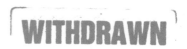

Diagnostic Imaging *for* Physical Therapists

Diagnostic Imaging
for Physical Therapists

James Swain, MPT
Director, Rehabilitation Services
Mercy Medical Center
Nampa, Idaho

Kenneth W. Bush, MPT, Ph.D.
Professor
Pacific University
School of Physical Therapy
Hillsboro, Oregon

With *a contribution by*:
Juliet W. Brosing, BSc, MSc, Ph.D.
Professor of Physics, Department Chair
Pacific University
Forest Grove, Oregon

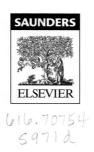

SAUNDERS

ELSEVIER

SAUNDERS

ELSEVIER

11830 Westline Industrial Drive
St. Louis, Missouri 63146

Notice

Neither the Publisher nor the Authors assume any responsibility for any loss or injury and/or damage to persons or property arising out of or related to any use of the material contained in this book. It is the responsibility of the treating practitioner, relying on independent expertise and knowledge of the patient, to determine the best treatment and method of application for the patient.

The Publisher

Vice President and Publisher: Linda Duncan
Executive Editor: Kathy Falk
Senior Developmental Editor: Christie M. Hart
Publishing Services Manager: Julie Eddy
Project Manager: Marquita Parker
Design Direction: Paula Catalano

Working together to grow
libraries in developing countries

www.elsevier.com | www.bookaid.org | www.sabre.org

ELSEVIER   BOOK AID International   Sabre Foundation

Printed in the United States

Last digit is the print number: 9 8 7 6 5 4 3 2 1

To my wife Linda who has been more tolerant of the time devoted to this effort than any husband has reason to expect. I am dearly thankful for all her advice and always graceful indulgence.

To my friend, colleague and co-author Ken Bush, PhD. who has been the vision, discipline, coordinator, and workhorse on this project. Without Dr. Bush this project simply would not have come to fruition.

James Swain

To all of my family: to my late mother, Velma who always assumed that I could do anything; and most especially, my wife Debbie who always makes my dreams her own; To my five children who have always made be proud to be their dad; To my PT students who make my job fun; and finally,

To Jim Swain, master clinician and gifted teacher, who had the foresight to collect interesting cases during his clinical career and then to convert his knowledge into information that the rest of us can use. It has been my privilege to sit in on his radiology courses with my students the past 10 years and to collaborate with him in creating this book.

Kenneth W. Bush

Preface

As Jim has traveled throughout the country teaching radiology courses, most therapists expressed inadequacy in reviewing and integrating imaging into their clinical practices at even a very basic level. Through the years, Jim evolved his radiology and imaging courses to give clinicians the knowledge and confidence that they needed to begin to use imaging in their practice.

This book is the culmination of Jim's experience and expertise in teaching radiology to students and clinicians throughout the United States. This book is an introduction to medical imaging and demonstrates a systematic methodology for reviewing medical imaging that will be helpful for clinical physical therapists as well as graduate students.

This volume also includes a DVD. The DVD contains numerous features helpful in developing imaging skills. The images are larger than can be printed in the book. It also contains animated, narrated views of standard x-ray images which will help develop a systematic method for reviewing diagnostic images.

We hope that this book will provide a deeper understanding of pathologies and further enhance your treatment planning and patient care.

James Swain
Kenneth W. Bush

Acknowledgments

This book acknowledges a number of colleagues and friends who have contributed over the years to our profession by their continued insistence on professionalism, evidence based practice, and vision for the future. I would be remiss if Betty Lambertson, Beth Hamilton, Joann Gronley, and Annie Webb, were not mentioned. They, and many other Army Medical Specialist Corps (AMSC) Officers helped shape the future direction of the physical therapy profession.

During the Vietnam War era, others in the AMSC, such as David Greathouse and Rick Ritter clearly saw the future of the physical therapy profession. 'Vision 2020' was put into practice in military physical therapy decades before it was articulated by our American Physical Therapy Association (APTA).

In the 1960's a young soldier returning from Viet Nam went to medical school and specialized in radiology. Dr. Robert 'Bob' Karl became one of the most generous and vocal physician advocates for the PT profession, and gave it professional recognition. He was among the first to give PT's clinical privileges to order and read x-ray films. The rules and disciplines learned by those of us privileged to know and work with Dr. Karl, became the bedrock of our beginnings in imaging.

Other highly respected and influential physicians include: Bruce Wheeler, Keith Markey, John Ryan, Robert Arciero, Jim Wheeler, and Jack McBride. All were evidence-based physicians who shared their knowledge, and gave their support without hesitation.

Several excellent images for our text were possible through the generosity of Drs. Kevin Shea and Andrew Curran; and their support is greatly appreciated.

Dr. Daiva Banaitis, formerly the director of the school of physical therapy at Pacific University supported and encouraged us in this project.

Dr. Juliet Brosing of the Pacific University department of physics has given lectures to our physical therapy class to help them understand the science of diagnostic imaging. She kindly agreed to author the chapter on the physics of medical imaging.

Michael Geraci and his crew at Pacific University who caught the vision of the multimedia DVD that we needed and worked long hours to create it.

In this same spirit of professional sharing and growth, we wish to acknowledge all who have made this book possible and hope that it will be an asset to the physical therapy profession.

James Swain
Kenneth W. Bush

Table of Contents

1 Introduction

INTRODUCTION TO THE BOOK

How This Book Is Organized

Chapter 1 is an introduction to how this book is organized and to the subject of medical imaging. This chapter is helpful in understanding how and why various forms of medical imaging are used.

Chapter 2 demonstrates a standardized method that can be used when viewing x-ray films. It is necessary to understand the rest of the book.

Chapter 3 is a review of the physics of medical imaging

Chapters 4 through 10 cover regions of the musculoskeletal system. They may be read in any order or be used individually as a reference when referring to plain film x-rays.

Chapter 11 is an introduction to magnetic resonance imaging (MRI). The chapter deals primarily with MRI images of the knee, but the concepts can be applied to MRIs of the other musculoskeletal regions of the body.

DVD Instructions

Medical imaging is a visual skill. To assist you in developing this skill, this book has an accompanying DVD which contains many additional features:

1. Standard views. Animations will show you how each standard view is taken.
2. Alignment, Bone density and dimension, Cartilage and Soft Tissue (ABCS). Video demonstrations will demonstrate how to use a standardized approach to review x-ray films for each body region and view.
3. Images. All x-ray films in the book are accessible at a higher resolution on the accompanying DVD.
4. Pathologies. For each body region being covered, common pathologies can be selected for comparison to normal films.
5. Case studies. Case studies are presented that allow you to apply your knowledge in determining what is causing the patient's complaints and in planning the treatment program.
6. Quizzes. Quizzes are available for each chapter. Each time you take a quiz, a different set of questions will be asked from a question bank.

When you see a **DVD** symbol 🔘 in the book, there is a feature available on the DVD. Start the DVD, go down the column on the left to the chapter that you are reading, and then select the feature across the top that you wish to use.

INTRODUCTION TO THE SUBJECT OF DIAGNOSTIC IMAGING

Diagnostic imaging for physical therapists has its genesis in military practice during the latter years of the Vietnam War. The lethality of the modern battlefield combined with the tremendous advances in battlefield evacuation by air, required vastly improved training for first responders (military aid men—the heroic "Medics"), and the upward spiral in quality of medical knowledge, surgical procedures, and trauma care led to the survival of badly wounded soldiers in heretofore unheard of numbers. This mandated that orthopedic surgeons spend more time in the operating suites and less time in the day-to-day outpatient clinics stateside and outside the war zone. Most general medical officers were not well trained in diagnosis and treatment of the orthopedic injuries generated in basic and advanced training of conscripted soldiers.

The military's answer was to place physical therapists in the troop medical clinics to do what was called "musculoskeletal screening.[1]" A portion of the credentialed privileges for these care providers was to order and read plain film x-rays to assist in ruling out fractures, significant soft tissue injuries, and joint instabilities. The films were also read by a radiologist as a backup before being returned to the nearest medical facility or hospital.

Musculoskeletal training programs worked well. In one study, physical therapists in primary care reduced imaging by 50% and patient acceptance was high.[1] This was the springboard for improving the skill of image interpretation for the profession of physical therapy. One recent study based upon an electronic review of 560 patients referred for MRI imaging in an 18 month period demonstrated that the clinical diagnostic accuracy (CDA) of physical therapists was significantly greater than nonorthopedic providers and that physical therapists are capable of making good clinical judgments regarding the ordering of diagnostic imaging studies and the diagnosis of musculoskeletal conditions independent of physician referral.[2]

Physical therapy has grown along with the rest of the healing professions in education, knowledge, and public recognition. Thirty years ago there were just a few entry level master's curricula in physical therapy. Now most of the professional curricula have, or are transitioning to, the 3-year graduate program with an entry-level doctorate. The profession now offers opportunities for the practitioner to achieve certification as a clinical specialist in a number of specialties and multiple postprofessional training fellowships are available to clinicians throughout the country and the world.

Imaging as an adjunct to practice has only recently begun to be taught and recognized within our profession via continuing education courses and in entry-level doctorate physical therapy programs. These students are taught the use of evidence-based clinical decision making in arriving at a physical therapy diagnosis and designing a successful treatment program.

There are few volumes written about imaging with focus on therapists and rehabilitation specialists. This book is written primarily: (1) to act as an introductory volume to establish a basic understanding of the various techniques of imaging as they exist today with an emphasis on standard, two-dimensional x-ray images; (2) to provide the therapist with a "systematic" basis for approaching the interpretation of standard films; and (3) to briefly introduce the more advanced techniques of imaging. It is *not* intended to be an all encompassing reference. Multiple volume references are already in existence. A few of the best known and most comprehensive are *The Diagnosis of Bone and Joint Disorders* by Drs. Donald Resnick and Gen Niiwayama,[3] *Orthopedic Radiology* by Dr. Adam Greenspan[4] and *Fundamentals of Orthopedic Radiology* by Lynn McKinnis.[5]

PHYSICAL THERAPY DIAGNOSIS

A correct and complete diagnosis is critical to the optimal provision of care. All interactions with the patient from the history and physical examination are combined with any other available information—including, but not limited to, movement analysis, laboratory studies, and imaging—to arrive at a working differential and physical therapy diagnosis. A working understanding of the potential causes of diseases of the musculoskeletal system is critical to successful understanding of imaging.

The purpose of the diagnosis according to the American Physical Therapy Association is to guide the therapist in determining the most appropriate intervention strategy for each patient/client.[6] In the event that the diagnostic process does not yield an identifiable cluster, syndrome, or category, intervention may be guided by the alleviation of symptoms, and remediation of deficits.[6]

A mnemonic that provides a quick review of other possible causes of abnormalities is the word *vindicate:*[7]

Vascular
Infection
Neoplasm
Drugs
Inflammatory/idiopathic
Congenital
Autoimmune
Trauma
Endocrine/metabolic

In addition to the individual clinical information supplied by imaging studies, this discipline provides the clinician with a vastly enhanced understanding and appreciation of the multiplanar relationships within the anatomical systems of the human body. Clinical examples are included as indicated to enhance teaching points. For example, one of the rules empha-

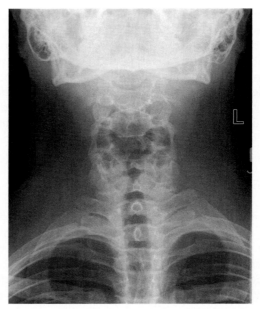

Figure 1-1. ■ **AP view of a normal cervical spine.** Note that the bifid spinous processes are aligned vertically, the trachea is midline, the lateral margins of the vertebrae are aligned. This view exposes only the lower cervical vertebrae, explaining the necessity for an "open mouth view" for the upper two cervical vertebrae.

sized in this book for the interpretation of standard two-dimensional x-rays is, "Some of the most important things you see, you cannot see." What this means, of course, is that what you can visualize on the standard x-ray are the effects these radiologically invisible lesions have on the surrounding skeletal structures and/or the reaction of the skeletal system to them. For example, a 21-year-old college athlete referred to physical therapy for shoulder strengthening and shoulder/neck pain arrives with a diagnosis of a "stinger" that he attributes to a tackle football game several months previous to his referral to the Physical Therapy Clinic. Four views of the patient's cervical spine may be seen in Figures 1-1 through 1-3. Normally, this represents a neuropraxia or axonotmesis—rarely a neurotmesis. A neuropraxia will most often resolve with time. In this case, the patient continued to have progressive weakness and pain in spite of repeated referrals back to the referring physician. Review of the standard x-ray series revealed an enlarged intervertebral foramen at the sixth and seventh cervical vertebral interface on

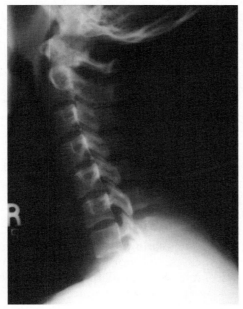

Figure 1-2. ■ This is a lateral view of a 21-year-old male college student referred to physical therapy with a "stinger." The patient was noted to have left-sided weakness at the C7 level. Note on this view the increased space at the C7 intervertebral foramen (just anterior to the articular facets) compared with the segment levels above. The change may seem subtle but when coupled with the clinical findings and the oblique views, the diagnosis becomes evident.

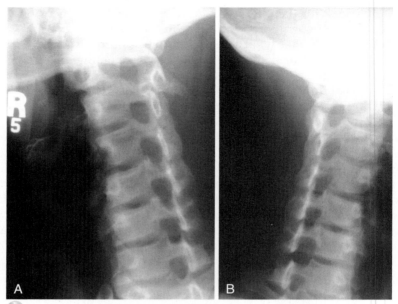

F*igure* 1-3 A *and* B. ■ The oblique on the R side demonstrates normal alignment and equal intervertebral foramen. The oblique on the L (the L marker was cropped) demonstrates the significant increase in size of the C7 nerve root when compared with the segments superior and inferior and to the same level on the R side. A schwannoma of the L C7 nerve root that had "jacked" the foramen open and was strangling the nerve root as it grew. The plain film does not show the tumor, but the result of the growth of the tumor is evident.

the same side as the weakness and pain. The patient had a schwannoma in the nerve root of C 6-7. On plain film views, the schwannoma was not visible, but clinically the increasing pain and weakness correlated exactly with the location of the increased opening at the appropriate cervical level. The schwannoma was strangling the nerve root and "jacking" the intervertebral foramen open as it grew. The treating therapist did not order the initial films in this case, and in most cases, will not need to order films. They may have been already taken and are usually available for viewing by asking. In those cases where the clinician feels he/she requires films to continue with the therapeutic intervention, a request to the referring physician may be all that is required.

Successful Treatment Planning

Anything that contributes to the correct diagnosis enhances the quality of care that the patient receives. The practice of treating the symptoms is tantamount to navigation without a compass.

When, for example, we evaluate a patient's back pain that includes a palpable lack of mobility at a specific segment, how are we to understand the cause of the immobility without further imaging? The immobility could be from myriad causes: failure of segmentation such as hemisacralization of L5-S1, severe arthritic changes, a space-occupying lesion, muscle spasm, or facet dysfunction. Clearly, hemisacralization or failure of complete segmentation would rule out manual therapy as a treatment option.

EVIDENCE-BASED CLINICAL DECISION MAKING

Patient care is improved with evidence-based clinical decision making. This is supported by data from multicenter studies, and studies using meta analysis.

Centers for Medicare & Medicaid Services (CMS) and managed care programs demand, and are entitled to, care based on clinically tested and proven regimens that have demonstrated the efficacy of specific treatment regimens and techniques. Imaging allows the clinician to "see" into the body. It is, however, a very selective type of sight based upon an understanding of multiple sciences including: physics, chemistry, physiology, biochemistry, mathematics, anatomy, and quantum mechanics, just to name a few.

The existing medical model system is built to protect the requesting clinician because the films are normally read by a radiologist as well as the clinician. Some clinicians are comfortable with just the written report, but tremendous information is often available on the films for the treating therapist that may not be mentioned in the dictated report. For example, the physician writing the initial request for the images may be interested in the patient's intervertebral disc at a specific level in the cervical spine as the etiology of the patient's referred pain, but the therapist may wish to know about the severity of accompanying degenerative changes, malalignment, and osteoporosis before undertaking a manual technique or designing the intensity of the therapeutic exercise program. As another example, the physician may refer the patient to therapy to initiate weight bearing following a fracture. The phrase, "Initiation of weight bearing" allows for an enormous amount of interpretation depending upon such variables as time from injury, time from surgical stabilization, the health of the individual's musculoskeletal systems, and other co-morbidities such as diabetes, advanced age, and medications, such as prednisone or other medications that could adversely affect their healing time. Therapists have at their disposal numerous tools in the clinic to control the level of weight bearing and/or stress on bones. The "Total Gym" can be adjusted based upon the patient's weight and the angle of inclination to allow for various levels of weight bearing, as can the horizontal shuttle. The latter is adjusted by increasing or decreasing the number of elastic bands the patient presses against while horizontally positioned on a sliding backrest. The important point is that these are day to day clinical decisions for the therapists that may require full understanding

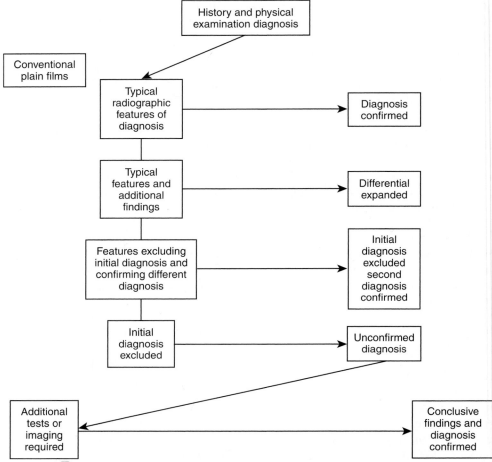

Figure 1-4. ■ An example of a decision-making matrix for integrating imaging into the evaluation of a patient referred for physical therapy. If additional imaging is indicated, the referring physician needs to be notified immediately.

of the status of the patient's musculoskeletal system and the specific anatomic status of this system. An example of a decision algorithm based on symptoms and signs from a patient with unilateral lumbosacral pain is shown in Figure 1-4.

It is worth mentioning that in 30 plus years of practice in military and civilian venues, the authors have encountered resistance from a physician to view or request information about a specific patient's imaging only once or twice. The vast majority of our physician colleagues are supportive and welcome another clinician's request to improve their understanding of the patient's condition to produce a positive outcome for the patient. There should never be a competition, or a second guessing of the medical diagnosis, but a collaborative attempt to gain information for the good of the patient. There are examples of another set of eyes and brain seeing a questionable density on the x-ray and referring the patient back to the physician to improve the patient's care.[8] With the exception of Chapter 3: The Physics of Medical Imaging and Chapter 11: An Introduction to MRI, this book will only touch superficially on the physics and mechanics of image production. To be true to the focus of this text and for brevity's sake, it is assumed that the undergraduate preparation of the therapist has provided a basis of understanding for these concepts.

CATEGORIES OF IMAGING

Reflective Imaging

Ultrasound and Magnetic Resonance Imaging (MRI)

Ultrasound and magnetic resonance imaging (MRI) are examples of reflective imaging. Energy is inserted into the system, captured, and converted into an image when it is returned. Ultrasound is a form mechanical compression of molecules, and MRI is a combination of electromagnetic and radio energy combined to produce signals from the body that can be collected and analyzed to produce an image.

Ionizing Radiation Imaging

Standard x-rays (standard or plain films), digital x-rays, and computed tomography (CT) require ionizing radiation exposure with its attendant risks.

Computed tomography is a form of ionizing radiation that uses the physical nature of ionizing radiation to penetrate matter and create a collectable image through the power of a computer. It is capable of producing an image or "slice" as narrow as 3 mm thick. It can be angled to analyze axially, coronally, sagittally, and tangentially. The software converts the x-rays that penetrate the body to Hounsfield units. These represent over 2000 levels of specificity between black and white. Water is the zero point with air at negative 1000 and metal at positive 1000. CT is recognized as the imaging of choice for evaluating bony pathology, whereas MRI is the imaging of choice for soft tissue pathology.

Emission Imaging

A bone scan is an example of emission imaging. Blood is drawn and tagged with a radiopharmaceutical agent, reintroduced to the body, and allowed to circulate throughout the entire body. As the radiopharmaceutical agent decays, it emits γ-rays. Over a short period of time, the areas of the body with increased metabolic activity—increased circulation—emit greater concentrations of the γ-rays. After sufficient time, usually 2 or 3 hours, the body is scanned with a scintillation camera to collect the γ emissions and produce an image that demonstrates areas of increased metabolic activity. A bone scan is binary; it is a yes or no answer. It tells you if an area demonstrates increased metabolic activity but not what is causing the increased metabolic activity. Scans are nonspecific and not diagnostic. As with all other forms of imaging, when combined with the history, examination, labs, etc., the bone scanning techniques may help confirm a diagnosis, but it is not diagnostic by itself. It is very helpful for identifying occult injuries to the skeletal system, demonstrating degenerative changes and for documenting the extent of certain metastatic lesions. It is very time sensitive and will be positive in the case of certain fractures, such as early overuse and/or stress syndromes or scaphoid fractures, before standard/conventional x-rays are positive. It can be very helpful in defining the extent of metastatic disease; information that can be critically important in the design of a cancer patient's rehabilitation plan. In cases of compromised vascular supply, a bone scan can be diagnostic before other forms of imaging, as in early avascular necrosis of the hip. Bone scans are more expensive than standard films but significantly less expensive than CT or MRI.

STANDARD X-RAY FILMS

X-ray evaluation, also referred to as plain or routine film, is the most commonly used form of imaging and forms the cornerstone of imaging. It is a visual and interpretive discipline that, on the most basic level, follows a series of analytical steps (standard or routine series) to arrive at clinically relevant information about the existence or nonexistence of pathology. Visualization of anatomy from the observation of x-ray films is a skill that requires diligence and practice to learn and improve, and is based upon a thorough working knowledge of anatomy and spatial relationships within the human body. Plain films will occasionally allow the clinician to see with his or her mind the pathology that may not be visible, but creates boney displacement or reactions such as lesions in the surrounding skeletal structures.

X-ray Production

The Four Major Densities
1. Air

   Air is the most radiolucent and absorbs the least numbers of particles from the beam resulting in the darkest portion and/or most exposed area of the negative/film/plate (Figure 1-5, *A* and *B*). Air and/or gas is normally found in the body within the trachea, lungs, and the colon.
2. Fat

   Fat absorbs more of the beam than air or gas but less than the other densities. Air and fat are considered radiolucent (black on x-ray, greater

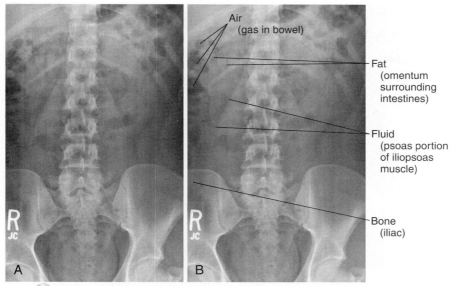

Air
(gas in bowel)

Fat
(omentum
surrounding
intestines)

Fluid
(psoas portion
of iliopsoas
muscle)

Bone
(iliac)

A   B

Figure 1-5 A and B. ■ AP lumbar spine without densities marked
(A); and with examples of densities marked (B).

film exposure because more x-ray energy is transmitted through these
media in the body to the film or cassette). Fat is found throughout the
body in amounts that vary between anatomical locations, individuals,
and genders. It is found from the subcutaneous tissue to the pericar-
dium and the omentum surrounding the intestines.

3. Fluid

   Fluid is more absorbent than air or gas and fat, and normally represents
   the varying densities of soft tissue organs and muscle. Fluid is of intermediate radiolucency. Note the psoas muscle outlined in Figure 1-5.

4. Bone

   Bone is the most dense, naturally occurring substance in the body.
   Calcium is the prime example of metal-like density found in the body.
   Calcifications and/or mineralization occur in nonbony locations of the
   body for various reasons. Examples are: myositis ossificans in muscle,
   pituitary mineralization in the base of the brain, aortic calcific deposi-
   tions, and renal calculi. Within bone itself there are obviously various
   densities. Cortical bone is much denser than cancellous bone. Per-
   ceived differences in images may depend upon the angle of exposure
   to the beam; as in an AP view of the scapula versus a lateral view of the
   same bone or an oblique view or AP view of the midshaft of the femur
   compared with an axial view. Bone is considered to be radio-opaque.

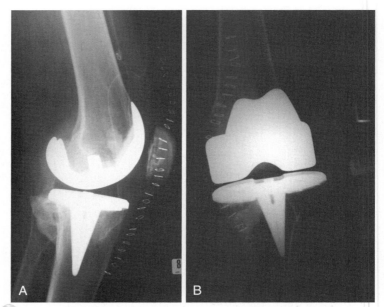

Figure 1-6 **A** *and* **B.** ■ Lateral **(A)** and AP **(B)** of a total knee arthroplasty (TKA). Surgery performed approximately 15 years prior to this image being taken.

Metal, such as metallic components of a joint arthroplasty; metallic internal fixation; fillings in teeth; and some remnants of trauma, such as bullets, shrapnel, etc.; are completely radio-opaque, the least radiolucent (Figure 1-6, *A* and *B*).

The orientation of the body part being x-rayed to the beam and the film cassette will determine the view that is produced. X-ray films can be taken with anterior/posterior, lateral, axial, tangential, sagittal, and oblique orientations. Figure 1-7 A and B demonstrates with a piece of plastic pipe (PVC) how the image is changed when a lateral view is contrasted with an axial view. In the same manner, these two views would change when x-ray film images are taken of a long bone from axial and lateral projections.

STANDARD VIEWS

Standard views, sometimes called routine views, are x-ray exposures that, by design and experience, have proven to be the optimal positional exposures to make a reasonable initial examination of a specific anatomical region or joint. The number of exposures required will vary from a minimum of two exposures taken at 90 degrees to one another, to cervical and lumbar spine series that require five exposures each. "One view is no view" is the rule that reinforces the

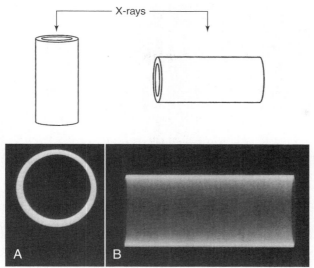

X-rays

A   **B**

🔵 **Figure 1-7 A *and* B.** ■ Radiographs made of a hollow plastic pipe from two different perspectives yield two entirely different images. The first image **(A)** reveals that the pipe is hollow but tells nothing about the length of the pipe. The second image **(B)** reveals the length dimensions of the pipe. Without having seen the first image, it is still possible to deduce that this object is tubular with a less dense center by observing the densities of the margins contrasting with the density of center. *(From Richardson and Iglarsh.* Clinical orthopedic physical therapy, *Philadelphia, 1994, WB Saunders.)*

requirement for a minimum of two views taken at 90 degrees to one another to provide a perspective on the position of potential pathology such as a fracture. A displaced oblique, distal tibial fracture may seem nondisplaced on the anterior/posterior view, but with the additional depth provided by the lateral projection and the mortise view, the fracture becomes obvious, with or without displacement (Figures 1-8 and 1-9).

An understanding of this concept is especially critical when evaluating increasing pain in a patient who has potentially reinjured a healing fracture, joint arthroplasty, or reports increased pain with an exercise that was not painful previously. Comparison films taken specifically to compare with the patient's most recent previous films or immediate postreduction films can be very informative. Figure 1-10 shows an example of a 25-year-old male patient who had sustained unilateral femur, tibial, and fibular fractures. While on a non-weight bearing, no driving restriction, he was cut off in an intersection while driving and slammed on the brakes with his injured leg. Immediately afterwards he noted an inability to extend his knee to complete extension as it had before this incident. In the views shown, there is a question about the position of the

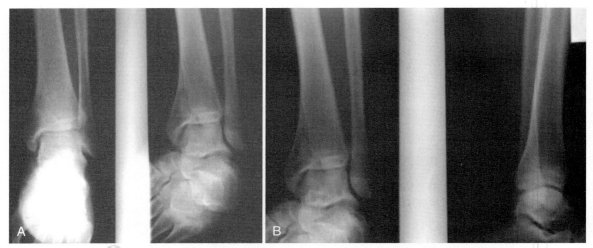

🔘 *Figure* 1-8 A *and* B. ■ **Three views of the ankle.** The AP and the lateral views are each shown next to the mortise view for comparison. The mortise view demonstrates a nondisplaced fracture of the medial, distal tibia that includes the plafond. This patient's rehab must not include weight bearing until the managing physician agrees to progressive weight bearing or until the fracture is stabilized surgically or demonstrates evidence of healing on the x-ray image.

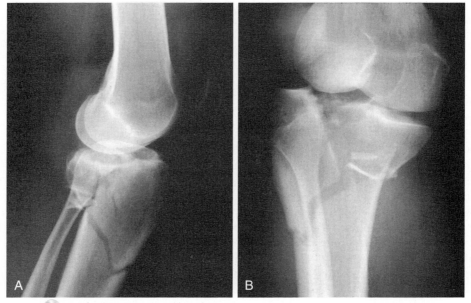

🔘 *Figure* 1-9 A *and* B. ■ AP and lateral of a 45-year-old female injured in a motorcycle/car accident: "One view is no view." The fractures, although clearly evident on the lateral view, do not reveal the extent of the fractures and the amount of displacement in the fracture until combined with the AP view to complete the assessment.

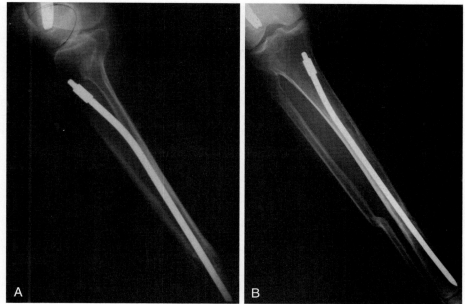

Figure 1-10 A *and* B. ■ A 25-year-old male after rod replacement of the femur and tibia reinjured leg with inappropriate weight bearing before being cleared for weight bearing by the surgeon. Immediate onset of pain with attempted full knee extension raised the question of traumatic migration distally of the femoral rod. Post "reinjury" films demonstrate that the rod has not migrated distally into the joint. The lateral view **(A)** is questionable but the AP **(B)** demonstrates that the rod is not into the articular surface. Comparison to pre "reinjury" films rules out the rod as the cause of the swelling and loss of motion.

femoral rod (see Figure 1-10). Has the rod moved distally into the joint? Is it the cause of his lost extension?

The answer is "No." After reviewing his previous films, taken before the traffic injury, and comparing them with his posttraffic injury films, it is clear that the rod has not moved. Additional information would be provided if the physician had requested films that demonstrated the entirety of the femoral rod throughout the femur. His loss of motion was due to the soft tissue trauma to the joint.

Body Position

The position of the body relative to the source of the x-ray beam and the "plate" or film are also of importance to the quality of the resultant x-ray exposure. Because photons and x-rays obey the physical laws of light, the shadows made with one's hands on a wall demonstrate the concept. The closer to the wall (plate or film) the object casting a shadow, the better the resolution of the shadow. The same holds true for an x-ray. Similarly, the further from the light source (x-ray beam source) the object casting the shadow is located, the more precise the resulting shadow (x-ray exposure). For example, if one were taking an x-ray of the lumbar spine, the ideal position would be with the patient lying supine with the film under the lower back and the source of the beam at the optimal length from the abdomen (Figure 1-11, *A-E*).

An x-ray is a two-dimensional negative with length and width. Your knowledge of normal anatomical relationships must supply that third dimension—depth, and the spatial relations in space—to what is essentially a two-dimensional relationship.

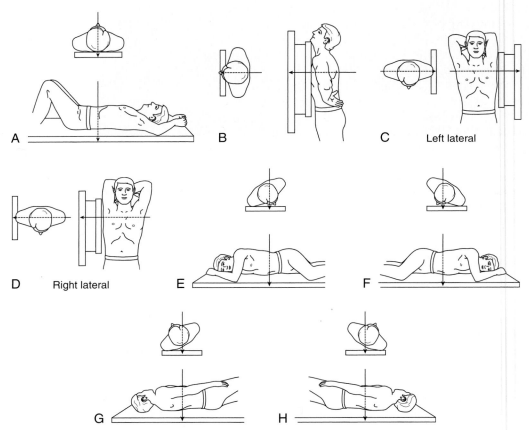

Figure 1-11 A-H. ■ **Patient positions for obtaining views of the spine.** **A,** AP, anteroposterior projection; **B,** PA, posteroanterior projection; **C,** Left lateral projection; **D,** Right lateral projection; **E,** PA oblique, right anterior oblique (RAO) position; **F,** PA Oblique projection, left anterior oblique (LAO) position; **G,** AP oblique projection, left posterior oblique (LPO) position; **H,** AP oblique projection, right posterior oblique (RPO) position. *(From Long BW, Frank ED, Ehrlich RA:* Radiography essentials for limited practice, *ed 2, Philadelphia, 2006, Saunders.)*

BASIC RADIOGRAPHIC PRINCIPLES[9]

A. "Do No Harm." The first principle of medicine applies here as well. Potential radiographic hazards include: genetic changes, bone necrosis, cancer, gonad damage, and damage to hematopoietic systems.

B. When written by the therapist, the radiographic request should be written clearly in standard terminology: Include a brief relevant history, physical findings, state what you want to x-ray, and describe the views. Help the radiologist help you.

C. Never use an x-ray as a substitute for taking a careful history and conducting a physical examination.

D. Correlate the history, physical findings, laboratory data, and x-rays to make an appropriate physical therapy diagnosis.

E. Avoid repetitious x-ray exposure and use shields for the gonads when possible to do so without compromising the view. The coned-down view of the lower lumbar spine produces an extremely high dose of radiation (rads) compared with other plain film exposures. The therapist should be very suspicious of significant lumbosacral pathology before requesting a coned-down view of the L5-S1 region. Is there another method of confirming the diagnosis? Will confirmation of the pathology with x-ray change the way you treat this patient?

F. Whenever history or examination/evaluation indicates the potential for a fracture, x-ray examination should be performed. Occasionally the patient will arrive in your clinic with symptoms and an examination that indicates that the pathology and/or injury was more significant than the referring physician may have suspected on the initial examination. A request to view the original films or a request for additional imaging before beginning treatment is entirely appropriate, particularly if it may change the treatment of the patient. A consultation with a colleague may be indicated. An example of this is an athlete with lateral foot pain assumed to be a stress reaction, which may in reality be a Jones fracture that will require an entirely different approach to care.
Never make an interpretation based on one view. Two views at right angles are the minimum required for proper interpretation. "One view is no view." With the AP view alone, we are unable to determine if the nail is in both the patella and the femur (Figure 1-12, *A*). However, the lateral view clearly shows that the nail in the distal femur is not through the patella and does not protrude through the posterior femur (Figure 1-12, *B*).

G. Include the joint above and below the suspected pathology. A patient with a low velocity, rotational torque fracture of the distal tibia may have an additional proximal fibular fracture, which is not an uncommon finding in a "ski boot" type fracture.

H. Lack of x-ray evidence of a fracture or abnormality does not rule out a fracture. The scaphoid bone, for example, often does not show plain film changes for up to 2 weeks from the fracture. If time is critical for decision making for the patient's care, a bone scan will be positive in 24 to 48 hours and at a cost that is one third of a CT or MRI.

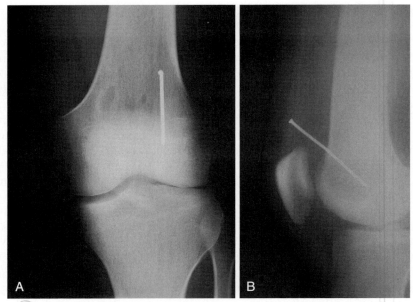

🌀 *Figure* 1-12 **A** *and* **B.** ■ A 28-year-old male construction worker who bumped his knee against the "working end" of a loaded nail gun while depressing the trigger with his index finger and other safety with his other fingers. The AP view alone leaves the question unanswered as to whether the nail includes the patella or the distance the nail has penetrated the femur **(A)**. The lateral view answers these questions **(B)**.

   I. Special studies may be indicated when signs or symptoms do not correlate with the x-ray findings (i.e., bone scan, CT scan, etc.)

   J. Soft tissue x-ray films can help rule out retained foreign bodies in lacerated or penetrating injuries.

  K. A view of both extremities, for comparison, may be required in certain instances; for example, young patients with open epiphyses that have a torsion injury.

  L. The frequency of follow-up x-rays depends upon various factors: the type of fracture, bones involved, age of the patient, and how the doctor is managing the patient's injury (i.e., open reduction internal fixation (ORIF) or casting) and the dependability and/or compliance of the patient.

  M. Suspected fractures not seen on an initial x-ray should be x-rayed again in 10 to 14 days or evaluated with further imaging studies. For example, a suspected fracture of the scaphoid bone in the wrist will not be visualized on plain films until demineralization of the peripheral regions of the fracture site is visible on the damaged bone.

  N. When an abnormality is found on x-ray, a differential diagnosis should include all possible diagnoses to be ruled out or accepted. The therapist's "index of suspicion" should be heightened when the patient's history does not reveal sufficient trauma or stress to have caused the injury visible on the image. The concern is always a preexisting disease that has weakened the skeletal system and predisposed the patient to injury.

O. All patients with a history of significant neck trauma should have a cross-table lateral of the cervical spine to rule out fracture or dislocation before any therapeutic intervention. This is important in diving accidents, surfing, body surfing, football injuries, motor vehicle accidents, falls, trampoline injuries, etc.

P. Postreduction films are required to judge the adequacy and maintenance of reductions. Always know your patient's status before therapeutic intervention.

Q. X-rays should be read on a view box and with a "hot light," not held up to a room light or ceiling light. In standard films of the shoulder, the subacromial region should be evaluated with the assistance of a "hot light." Calcification of the supraspinatus tendon shows best with this technique.

R. Procedures, such as arthrograms, carry the risk of infection and allergic reaction. Most of these techniques have been supplanted by MRI and CT.

S. Always view fractures, even with a history of trauma, with the suspicion of a pathological etiology: osteoporosis, metabolic disorders, genetic abnormalities, such as osteogenesis imperfecta, and primary or metastatic disease weaken bone.

T. Accept only quality x-rays. Underexposed or overexposed films are worse than a waste of time because they may lull you into a sense of false security. Although the vast majority of films taken within the last 10 years are of a standardized level of very high quality, there are still a few that originate in private practitioner's offices that do not meet accepted standards.

Question: Can you evaluate with certainty whether a shoulder is dislocated on the two standard views of the shoulder—AP and abduction/internal rotation view?

Answer: No. The majority of anterior dislocations of the shoulder show quite clearly on the standard AP view and abduction/internal rotation films mentioned above. However, when evaluating the shoulder, especially following trauma, it is mandatory to obtain an additional x-ray at right angles to the frontal x-rays to determine the relative positions of the humeral head and glenoid. This view is known as a trauma view or a transscapular view and demonstrates the position of the humeral head superimposed on the glenoid. This view shows the glenoid contained within the circumference of the humeral head, effectively ruling out a posterior dislocation. Additionally the "West Point" view assists with this evaluation.

ORIENTATION OF THE FILMS FOR INTERPRETATION

A. Check the patient's name on the film to ensure you have the correct films.

B. Check the dates so that the films can be viewed chronologically.

C. Orient the films correctly on the view box by date and sequence that you want to evaluate. Be consistent in the manner you read them.

    D. Check for the Right ("R") and Left ("L") markers.

    E. **Develop a system!** This is critical! Be consistent with your system. In standard views of x-ray films in the anterior/posterior and posterior/anterior projections, the film is always positioned so the projection is of the patient in the anatomic position as if the patient was facing you.[10]

    The x-ray findings are only a part of the evaluation. Always, in the absence of significant radiographic findings, base your assessment on clinical findings and not solely on the images, and account for all apparent inconsistencies before initiating a therapeutic intervention.

BONE DYNAMICS

Bone is specialized tissue that contributes multiple functions to the body. The endoskeleton functions to provide attachments to support the motor movements of the muscular system, protects many of the vital organs of the body, and houses the sites of hemopoiesis. Bone is dynamic living tissue that reacts to its environment by strengthening areas subjected to stress and demineralizing and eliminating areas that no longer provide functional structural support to the body. This process is described by "Wolff's law." Wolff's law is, arguably, the most functional concept for understanding bone's reaction to stress. Simply stated, stressed bone reacts over time by strengthening the areas of increased stress and demineralizing or eliminating the areas of lowered stress (stress shielding). Trabecular patterns develop along the lines of stress and stress fractures develop perpendicular to the trabeculae. Dr. Michael Richardson, from the University of Washington, paraphrases this by explaining that, "Bone reacts to its environment in two ways—either by removing some of itself or creating more of itself.[7]" The skeletal system that has weight-bearing stress significantly reduced, as in prolonged bed rest, or removed entirely, as in space travel, will become osteopenic. Localized immobilization, as seen in a non–weight-bearing, casted lower extremity may develop localized osteopenia. Bone reacts to its environment like any other tissue but in slow motion. Understanding this concept is critical to evaluating images of bone. A tibial fracture, if stabilized by plates and screws so completely that the bone bears no weight, will heal extremely slowly, if at all. The femoral component in a total hip arthroplasty (THA), if not placed so that the portion of the femur that transfers weight to the proximal femoral shaft femur bears weight in an even and/or normal fashion, may result in a demineralization in the proximal femur immediately below the area of the prosthesis where no stress is transmitted to the bone.

    The outer surface of bone is covered by the periosteum; a fibrous tissue of amazing strength. The periosteum is of such strength that it may, at times, be the only remaining restraining structure to hold the bone fragments in proximity during severe fracture. It is composed of two layers: the thick, tough fibrous layer and just below that, the cambium layer. This innermost layer of the cambium contains the osteoblasts, cells that assist with the healing of injured bone (Figure 1-13).

    Test your understanding by taking a quiz on this chapter with the accompanying DVD.

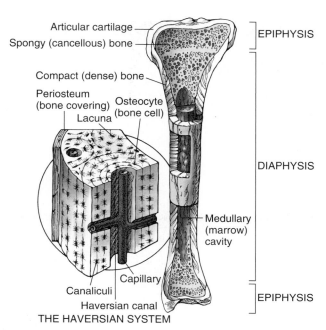

Articular cartilage
Spongy (cancellous) bone
EPIPHYSIS

Compact (dense) bone
Periosteum
(bone covering)
Osteocyte
(bone cell)
Lacuna

DIAPHYSIS

Medullary
(marrow)
cavity

Canaliculi
Capillary
Haversian canal
THE HAVERSIAN SYSTEM

EPIPHYSIS

Figure 1-13. ■ **The structure of the bone.** (*From Ignatiavicius, DD. Medical-surgical nursing: critical thinking for collaborative care, 5e, Saunders, Philadelphia, 2005*).

REFERENCES

1. Greathouse D, Schreck R, Benson C: The United States Army physical therapy experience: evaluation and treatment of patients with neuromusculoskeletal disorders, *JOSPT* 19:5, 261-266 1994.
2. Moore J et al: Clinical diagnostic accuracy and magnetic resonance imaging of patients referred by physical therapists, orthopaedic surgeons, and nonorthopaedic providers, *J Ortho & Sports Phys Ther* 35:2:67-71, 2005.
3. Resnick D, Niwayama G: *Diagnosis of bone and joint disorders,* ed 2, Philadelphia, 1998, WB Saunders.
4. Greenspan A: *Orthopedic radiology,* ed 2, New York, 1992, Raven Press.
5. McKinnis L: *Fundamentals of orthopedic radiology,* Philadelphia, 1997, F.A. Davis.
6. American Physical Therapy Association: Guide to Physical Therapy Practice, APTA, 1999, pp 1-7.
7. Richardson M: Approaches to differential diagnosis in musculoskeletal imaging. Sclerotic lesions of bone. *http://www.rad.washington.edu/mskbook/sclerotic.html.*
8. Carlton R, Adler A: Principles of radiographic imaging, ed 3 (Delmar, 2001) p 132.
9. U. S. Army training manual for radiology technicians, Headquarters, Dept. of the Army, 1971.
10. McKinnis L: Home study course, diagnostic imaging of bones and joints, introduction to the science of orthopedic radiology, APTA, Orthopedic Section, p 6.

2 Systematic Analysis Using ABCS

INTRODUCTION

Remarks

This chapter will demonstrate a systematic approach to evaluating an x-ray film for any part of the body. As you practice this system, you will become comfortable with the items that you will and will not see in typical x-ray films. As you correlate what you see on the films with what you see in the patient's physical exam, you should develop a better understanding of the patient's condition and the treatment that will be necessary to help the patient make maximal improvement.

This chapter will present a lateral view of the cervical spine as an example. The concepts that you learn in this chapter will be used throughout the book as we examine the body, joint by joint.

Each joint has specific views that have been developed to visualize the maximum number of structures. Each view should be considered using a systematic approach, which we will call the ABCS system. However, some of the system may not be used for a particular view. For example, a sunrise view of the knee is used to visualize the alignment of the patella with the femoral groove, but does not show the soft tissue of the knee in a useable way.

OBJECTIVES

1. Recall the four steps of a standardized x-ray film evaluation.
2. Identify normal and abnormal alignments of an x-ray film.
3. Identify normal and abnormal bone densities on an x-ray film.
4. Identify normal and abnormal bone dimensions on an x-ray film.

5. Identify normal and abnormal cartilage presentations on an x-ray film.

6. Identify normal and abnormal soft tissue presentations on an x-ray film.

SYSTEMATIC ANALYSIS OF PLAIN/ROUTINE X-RAY FILMS OF MUSCULOSKELETAL IMAGES

The most critical factor in successfully evaluating plain/standard/routine x-ray films is a disciplined, systematic analysis. This ensures that the critical structures are carefully viewed and analyzed in an orderly fashion that minimizes the tendency of the clinician to focus in on the preconceived "pathology" that he or she is leaning toward from their history and physical evaluation of the patient. One strength of our medical practice model is that it mandates that a radiologist evaluate all the films taken in the radiology department and generate a report unencumbered and unbiased by the complete history and physical examination. An effective system available to the novice for the evaluation of the musculoskeletal system is to apply the "ABCS" system, which stands for alignment, bone density and dimension, cartilage, and soft tissue.[1-4]

Alignment

Alignment in clinical radiology refers to one bone's relationship to the bones it is immediately connected to. It is critical to remember that almost all bony articulations are maintained by connective tissue. The assessment of alignment relates to stability and integrity of the bones and the connective tissues that maintain these critical relationships. Instability can occur as a result of trauma and fractures, connective tissue damage, or laxity caused by stretching, congenital anomalies, and acquired or inherent diseases.

The initial focus is toward the overall appearance of the structure(s) being analyzed and evaluated (Figure 2-1). Is the cervical spine lordotic, the thoracic spine kyphotic, and the lumbar spine lordotic? Specific lines are drawn mentally through anatomical points to assess these relationships. The bony region of assessment is evaluated for overall size, shape, and integrity: Are the cortical margins without breaks or interruptions, and are the articular relationships spatially maintained? Two views are the minimum required. In the spine, this includes the relative positions of the vertebral segments in relation to the adjacent segments. In the extremities, the joints and bones are evaluated by the positions of the articular portions of the bones relative to their adjacent articular surfaces. For example: Do the proximal humerus and the glenoid align on both the AP external rotation view and on the abduction, internal rotation view? If there is any doubt, a transscapular view can be requested. If there is a question of alignment in the spine or peripheral joints, there are "special views" to assess their alignment more specifically. These will be reviewed in each chapter.

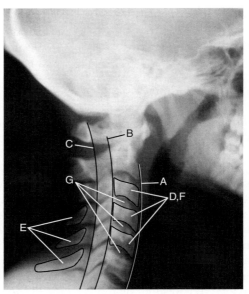

Figure 2-1. ■ **Lateral view of the cervical spine with alignment points identified. A**lignment: Anterior longitudinal ligament (ALL) line is smooth. Posterior longitudinal line is smooth. Spinous process laminar interface line is smooth. **B**one: Density is consistent among vertebral bodies and spinous processes. Dimensions are equal between vertebral bodies. **C**artilage: The disk spaces between vertebral bodies are equal. **S**oft tissue: Note the soft tissue anterior to the ALL. A = ALL; B = PLL; C = Spinous processes laminar interface line; D = Vertebral bodies; E = Spinous processes; F = Height of the vertebral bodies.

Bone

The health of the skeletal system is interconnected to the overall health of the organism through many interdependent physiologic feedback loops and chemical checks and balances. The health of the musculoskeletal system is one of the windows into the overall status of the entire organism.

Bone is evaluated in several general categories that are individually tailored to the specific anatomic regions being reviewed. Long bones are referred to by the region of the individual bone being evaluated and include: the diaphysis or shaft of the long bone, the metaphysis or flared transition from the diaphysis to the articular portion of the bone and the articular region of the bone referred to as the epiphysis. The architectural structure of bone follows the old adage that "form follows function." The long shafts of the extremity bones, the cortical bones, provide strength and are hollow to decrease weight. The epiphyses of these bones are widened to increase the articular surface and decrease the pressure on the surface area, but are made up of cancellous (spongy) bone that lessens the weight of this enlarged surface area.

Bone is evaluated in two major areas: bone density and bone dimension.

Bone Density

Density is specific to the anatomic portion of the skeletal system and to that portion of bone being imaged, along with the age of the patient and the existence of any co-morbidities. In the vertebral column, with a few notable exceptions, the segments above and below are good indicators of the appropriate density of the segment of interest. An obvious exception would be the first and second cervical segments whose densities and dimensions are atypical. However, as you move further distally in the spinal column, the transitions are much more gradual. In the extremities, the cortical bone should appear dense on the periphery and less dense along the medullary canal. The articular portion of the long bones from the metaphysis to the articular surface is composed of cancellous bone and should have consistent trabecular patterns throughout. Any inconsistency or abrupt change in these patterns, areas of increased or decreased density, or significant variation in the normal trabecular pattern should arouse suspicion, warrant further investigation, and be included in the clinician's differential list.

When reviewing the overall shape and integrity of the bone, the periosteum should be noted and evaluated for any swelling or "lifting" away from the bone. In healthy bone, the periosteum is tightly adherent to the surface of the cortical bone. If it is elevated from the bone, it indicates a pathologic change in its normal relationship to the cortex. Examples of causes of this elevation from the bone are: swelling from death of small portions of the bone from sickle cell sludging, periosteal lifting by the callous formation of an incipient stress fracture, displacement of the periosteum from tumor growth or space occupying lesion, and subperiosteal hemorrhage.

Bone Dimensions

Dimensions in the systematic evaluation of plain/routine x-rays are specific to the anatomic region and bone being evaluated. For example, the spinal segments immediately above and below the area of interest are excellent indicators of the appropriate dimensions of the segment being studied, whereas the extremities are evaluated for dimensions that are typical or "within normal limits." These dimensions are quickly learned with practice reading x-ray films. Comparison views that evaluate one side with respect to the other can be helpful if the other extremity is not involved. These specific dimensions will be reviewed with each anatomic region. There are specific endocrine, physiologic, and nutritional pathologies that result in abnormal shapes and sizes of bone. For example: Hypersecretion of growth hormone from the pituitary during the growth period will produce a tall person, and this same hypersecretion after the epiphyseal plates are closed will result in a condition known as acromegaly. This latter condition can be mimicked by body builders who take growth hormone as a supplement to their training regimens. An individual with Marfan syndrome, a connective tissue disease, can have extremely long extremities, and fingers and toes; a condition referred to as arachnodactyly.

Cartilage

The intervertebral discs in the spine and the articular surfaces of the synovial joints are composed of cartilage. Cartilage can be viewed as a "spacer" between bony articular surfaces. In the spine and extremities, the bones demonstrate decreased distance between the articular surfaces, especially in weight-bearing joints as the cartilage is worn away or after it is removed. In the extremities, the "cartilage" portion of the systematic evaluation will include hyaline/articular cartilage and meniscal or labral fibrocartilage. Tears in the articular hyaline and fibrocartilaginous structures are not normally visible on plain x-rays without special procedures, such as an arthrogram, but their absence or damage can eventually take their toll on the health of the bone in proximity to them and result in radiologically recognizable changes to that bone. A knee joint without the benefit of the cushioning, lubricating, and spacing of the medial meniscus will gradually shift into varus or valgus and often wear out the remaining hyaline cartilage, resulting in characteristic arthritic changes in the articular surfaces of the femur and tibia. Eventually,

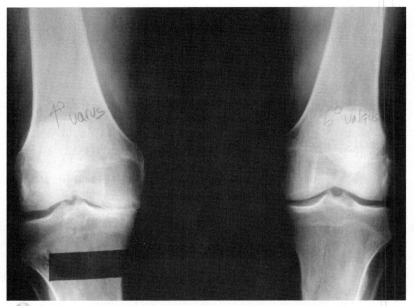

Figure 2-2. ■ **AP views of both knees.** The knee on the left as you view these films is in increased varus and the medial femoral condyle is "bone on bone" with the medial tibial plateau. Note the lack of joint space, the flattening of the medial femoral condyle and the increased density of the bones in contact. This increased density is characteristic of "bone on bone" degeneration.

the bone-on-bone abrasion will result in a thickening of the contact surfaces seen on plane/routine films as an increased density or "whitening of the bone." This condition, along with an accompanying varus or valgus and loss of joint space, is diagnostic of a knee without the protection of meniscal cartilage (Figure 2-2).

A spinal segment without the cushioning and space maintenance of the nucleus will gradually collapse onto the segment below with recognizable degenerative changes to the surrounding bony structures and malalignment of the distal articular facets (Figure 2-3).

Soft Tissue

Soft tissue is evaluated because it affects the musculoskeletal system. A systematic approach to evaluating the spine and joints of the musculoskeletal system requires a critical review of the soft tissue that is visible in the area being studied. The visible portion of the lung should be scanned for changes in consistency or displacement while reviewing shoulder and neck films. Any displacement of the trachea as seen on an AP view of the cervical spine may indicate

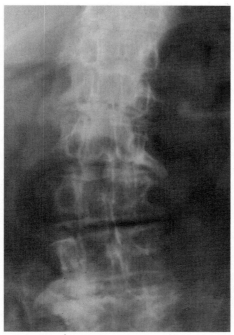

Figure 2-3. ■ **AP of the lumbar spine with scoliosis, severe degenerative changes, demineralization, and osteophytosis.** Note the decreased joint space at multiple levels.

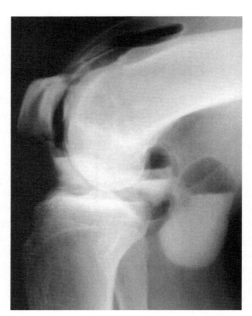

Figure 2-4. ■ **Lateral view of an arthrogram of the knee.** The extent of the synovial system in the knee, the largest and most extensive in the body, is evident in this x-ray film of a Baker cyst. The differential diagnosis possibilities for a lump in the posterior knee might include: Baker cyst, tumor, popliteal aneurysm, etc. The arthrogram confirms the cyst. An MRI would also confirm the diagnosis and is noninvasive.

pressure from a space occupying lesion, a pneumothorax or a hemothorax. Any inconsistency in the density of the surrounding muscle tissue should be noted and explored via the referring physician or radiologist. Margins of the joint space and soft tissue surrounding the joint should be assessed for swelling and soft tissue displacement (Figure 2-4).

Test your understanding by taking a quiz on this chapter with the accompanying DVD.

REFERENCES

1. McKinnis L: Fundamentals of orthopedic radiology, Philadelphia, 1997, FA Davis.
2. Forrester D: The radiology of joint disease, ed 2, Philadelphia, 1978, WB Saunders.
3. Daffner RH: Clinical radiology: the essentials, Baltimore, 1993, Williams & Wilkins.
4. Swain JH: An introduction to radiology of the lumbar spine: orthopedic study course 94-1 APTA, 1994.

3 The Physics of Medical Imaging

Juliet W. Brosing

INTRODUCTION

This chapter is designed to give a basic understanding of the science behind the imaging techniques described in this book. A fundamental knowledge of how the different imaging systems work and the limitations of the different types of imaging is vitally important to your service to your patients. Because many patients spend more time with their therapists, they are often inclined to ask questions of the physical therapist that they would not necessarily ask their doctor. The information in this chapter is intended to help you interpret your patients' medical images and respond to questions that patients may have.

This chapter will discuss x-rays and the sophisticated computed tomography (CT) scans, bone scans, and magnetic resonance imaging (MRI). The majority of the discussion will be about MRIs, both because they are much more complicated and because they are of such valuable use to PTs.

X-RAYS AND CT SCANS

X-ray images are essentially a shadow, a projection image, which creates a two-dimensional image from a three-dimensional body. X-rays are directed at the patient. A film or other type of receptor is placed behind the patient. When this is exposed, the shadow on the film indicates where the x-rays were absorbed, thereby revealing breaks in the bone structure, etc. The shades of gray on a

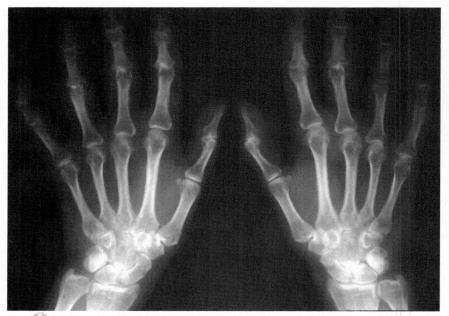

Figure 3-1. ■ Standard x-ray of hands, showing detail of bone structure.

diagnostic x-ray represent varying absorption of the x-rays. Figure 3-1 shows an x-ray of hands. Notice the detail of the bones.

X-rays are excellent for indicating broken bones since the difference in absorption of x-rays between bones and soft tissue is large. Thus, if a bone is broken, the x-rays "get through" and expose the receptor, clearly indicating a break. This can be seen in Figure 3-2 where a fracture of the proximal ulna is clearly visible.

Production of X-rays

X-rays are a form of electromagnetic energy. They are part of the electromagnetic spectrum shown in figure (Figure 3-3). Other parts of the electromagnetic spectrum you may be more familiar with include visible light, microwaves, ultraviolet light, etc. All the parts of the electromagnetic spectrum are uncharged, transverse waves that travel at the speed of light. Because the electromagnetic energy is neutral in charge, and has no mass, it interacts very little with the material it goes through. A "packet" of electromagnetic energy is referred to as a photon. (Don't get this confused with protons in the nucleus. A proton is positively charged and has a mass; a photon is neutral and is pure energy without mass.) The characteristic that differentiates the various types of radiation in the electromagnetic spectrum shown in Figure 3-3 is the energy (and thus the wavelength) of the radiation. X-rays and γ-rays have much higher energy (and much shorter wavelength) than other parts of the electromagnetic spectrum.

A point of confusion for some is the distinction between gamma rays and x-rays. As you can see from the electromagnetic spectrum figure their energies

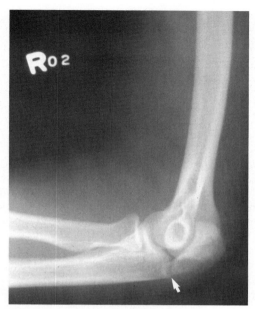

Figure 3-2. ■ **X-ray of the elbow.** A fracture of the proximal ulna is evident (*arrow*).

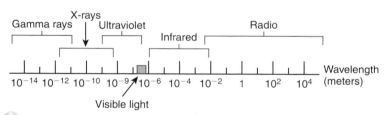

Figure 3-3. ■ **Electromagnetic spectrum.** Gamma rays have the shortest wavelength and thus the highest energy. All types of electromagnetic radiation are transverse waves that travel at the speed of light. Differences in properties are due to the differences in wavelength (and thus energy and frequency).

overlap. Basically gamma rays are created in the nucleus and x-rays are created at the atomic level. Thus x-rays are usually created by accelerated electrons hitting a target, and gamma rays are emitted from radioactive nuclei. However the important point is that they both are used in imaging and the results are the same.

The creation of x-rays is quite simple but ingenious. See Figure 3-4 for a schematic of an x-ray tube.

A source of electrons is created by a heated cathode (see C in Figure 3-4) that "boils" electrons off a filament (see F in Figure 3-4). The electrons are then accelerated across a large potential difference until they are moving very fast.

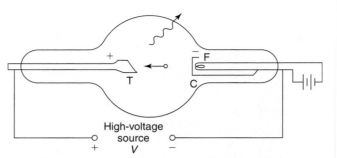

■ **Figure 3-4.** ■ **X-ray tube.** A high voltage source creates a large potential difference between the cathode (C) and the anode (T). Electrons are "boiled" off the heated cathode and accelerate towards the anode because of this potential difference. When they reach the anode (T), they abruptly stop. This change in momentum and energy creates the x-rays.

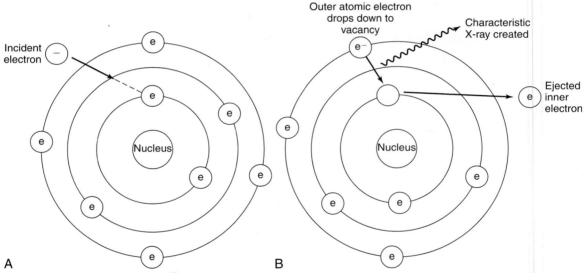

■ **Figure 3-5.** ■ **Characteristic x-ray production. A,** Atomic electrons are orbiting about the nucleus. An energetic electron from the heated cathode collides with an inner atomic electron in the target, ejecting it from the atom. **B,** An atomic electron from an outer shell jumps down to the vacancy created in the inner shell. A characteristic x-ray, equal to the energy difference between the two shells, is created to conserve energy.

They then hit the positive metal anode T (usually Tungsten) and abruptly come to a stop. This creates two types of x-rays: specific discrete energies referred to as characteristic x-rays and a continuum of energies referred to as bremsstrahlung. The characteristic x-rays (as shown in Figure 3-5) are created by the electrons colliding with inner electrons in the atoms of the metal anode, giving them enough energy to leave the atom.

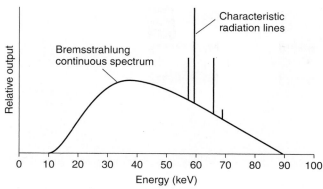

Figure 3-6. ■ **X-ray energy spectrum.** The broad spectrum of energies is due to the bremsstrahlung radiation and is used in medical imaging. The specific peaks are characteristic of the metal in the anode.

Then electrons in the outer shells drop down to these vacancies in the inner shells, and in doing so, emit characteristic x-rays with energy equal to the difference in the energy levels between the atomic electron shells. The bremsstrahlung (or "braking") radiation comes from an accelerated electron bypassing the atomic electrons and coming close to a nucleus in the target. Because of the interaction between the accelerated electron and the positive nucleus, the electron's kinetic energy is decreased. To conserve energy, a photon in the range of x-ray energies is emitted. The majority of the x-rays used in medical imaging are from bremsstrahlung radiation.

If you look at the energy distribution of the x-rays created, you will see, as shown in Figure 3-6, a broad spectrum of energies as a result of the bremsstrahlung radiation and specific peaks that represent the characteristic x-rays. If a different metal were used in the anode, there would be different energies of the characteristic x-rays.

Film/Screen Radiography

To create images, you need not only a source of x-rays but also a projection system. Two projection systems we will briefly discuss are screen-film radiography and digital radiography.

Screen-film radiography is the oldest imaging technique. The x-rays are transmitted into the patient's body; some are absorbed, and those that aren't are detected on the other side by the film-screen system.

Film by itself can be used to detect x-rays (that is how they were discovered), but it is relatively inefficient. It takes a large x-ray dose to provide a useful x-ray image on film. In modern radiography, screens are used together with film to improve the images and reduce the patient dose. The screen is made of a phosphor material that produces light when exposed to x-rays. The film and one or two intensifying screens are encased in a light-tight screen-film cassette (Figure 3-7).

Two important types of x-ray images are anteroposterior projection (AP) and posteroanterior projection (PA). In an AP image, the detector is behind (or

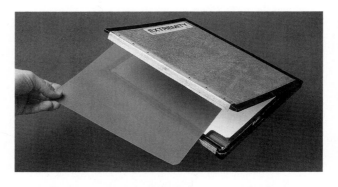

| Fluorescent Screen #2 |
| Film |
| Fluorescent Screen #1 |

Figure 3-7. ■ Image of screen/film cassette. The x-ray film is sandwiched between two fluorescent screens, which are all encased in a light-tight cassette. This improves the images and reduces patient dose. *(Top, from Frank ED:* Merrill's Atlas of Radiographic positioning and procedures, *11e, Mosby, St. Louis 2007)*

underneath) the patient, and the x-rays are coming through the front of the patient (Figure 3-8).

In a PA image, the chest is against the detector and the x-rays are coming through the back of the patient (Figure 3-9).

Anyone reading x-rays should be aware of distortions caused by the distance from the central beam. Ideally the x-ray beam and the image receptor should be perpendicular to the anatomical part one wishes to image. The farther the body part is from the central beam, the greater the distortion. (This is similar to observing shadows. If the light source is immediately behind the object, the shadow will be crisp and sharp. If the source is farther away, and at an angle, the shadow will be distorted.)

In muscular-skeletal imaging, the image being studied must be closest to the film/receptor to prevent edge blurring and/or penumbra effect. Figure 3-10, *A* shows an AP projection, where the spine is closest to the film. Note the detail of the spine. Figure 3-10, *B* is a PA projection, where the chest is closest to the detector. It shows better detail of the lungs. (Although both figures are of the same patient, Figure 3-10, *B* is 'higher up" since the goal was to see the lungs.) Figure 3-10, *A* is taken from the base of the spine, which is not evident in Figure 3-10, *B*. There is an area of dense calcification, which is seen as solid white near the top of

Detector   **X-rays**

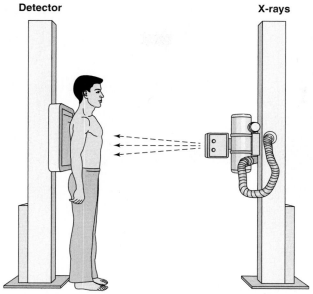

Figure 3-8. ■ **Schematic of AP projection.** The detector is underneath or behind the patient, and the x-rays are coming through the front of the patient.

X-rays Source   **Detector**

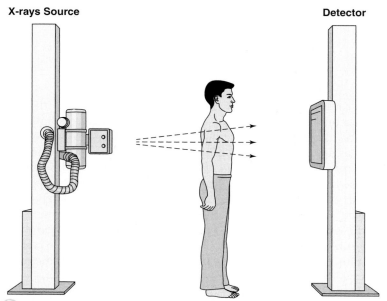

Figure 3-9. ■ **Schematic of PA projection.** The detector is in front of or above the patient, and the x-rays are coming through the back of the patient.

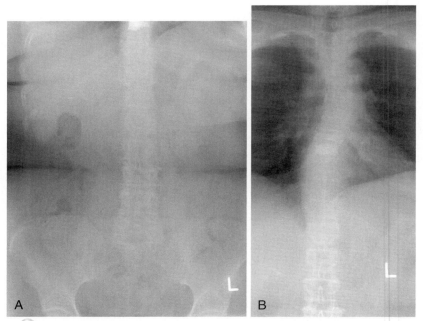

Figure 3-10. ■ **A**, An anterior to posterior (AP) view of the thoracic and lumbar spine. Note that the spinal column is in better focus than in **B**. **B**, A posterior to anterior (PA) view of the thorax. Note that the lung fields are more in focus with the spinal column less focused. The PA film is used to visualize the lungs, not the spine.

the image in Figure 3-10, *A* that shows up midway down the spine in Figure 3-10, *B*, which allows the viewer to orient the two images relative to one another.

Digital Radiography

With digital radiography the film/screen system is replaced with a digital receptor and an image processor. One of the big advantages of digital radiography is that the image processor can enhance and optimize the image after it is recorded. In addition, the storage of the digital image has many advantages: it requires less physical space, images can be rapidly retrieved and stored, and images can be duplicated without loss of image quality. Digital receptors have a much wider dynamic range than film. The number of increments in shading between black and white is much greater, so finer differences can be seen.

One of the challenges of digital radiography is knowing when the receptor is correctly and optimally exposed. On film it is obvious since if not done correctly, the film is underexposed or overexposed. In digital radiography, it is possible to overexpose the image of the patient but still get good contrast. In general, for a radiographic procedure there is an optimum exposure that produces a good balance between image noise and patient exposure. The challenge to the technologist is to make sure that the technique factors are set to produce this optimum exposure.[1]

Today most imaging techniques are digital. MRIs and CT scans only became possible because of the large computing power available and are digital images. Ultrasound and nuclear medicine images went digital in the 1970s. Radiography is the last important imaging technique to be converted to digital. Surprisingly, much more memory is required to digitize a typical x-ray than a typical MRI image. If x-rays are to be part of a digital imaging system throughout a hospital complex, much higher resolution screens and greater memory requirements are necessary. Thus it is enormously expensive to include x-rays as part of a digital delivery system. In this context, two acronyms you may come across are DIMS for digital image management system and PACS for picture archiving and communications system. Although the cost for such a digital delivery system is expensive, hospitals (especially in remote locations) can save money by implementing such a system and then "sharing" a radiologist at another location. The radiologist is basically on call, but doesn't have to be on-site to read the images.

X-rays are the oldest imaging modality and many advances have been made to the image quality. As you can see from many of the images in this text it is often possible to observe phenomenal detail of the inside of the human body, particularly of anatomical structure. X-rays are relatively inexpensive, readily available, quick to obtain, and are most often the modality of choice in the initial assessment of injury and disease.

X-rays are valuable not only for imaging but also for treatment. It is important to help your patients understand the difference between x-rays used as an imaging technique (e.g., for bone breaks) and x-rays used as a cancer treatment. Because cancer cells are rapidly dividing, they are sensitive to damage from radiation. With much greater concentrations of x-rays than those used for imaging, the x-rays can kill cancer cells.

CT Scans

Computed tomography (CT) combines multiple x-rays with the impressive computing power currently available to create tomographic images of the patient (Figure 3-11). X-rays are taken from many different angles and then sophisticated computer programs manipulate this data to create a digital image of a particular plane through the patient's body. CT scans are fast, relatively cheap, and widely available at most hospitals. They are not as good as MRIs for soft tissue injuries (although much better than a single x-ray)—because the difference in x-ray absorption between the injured and healthy tissue is often not significant enough to see on the detector. CT scans are often used in the chest and abdomen area, and originally were used a lot with brain images. MRI has since replaced the CT scan for most images of the brain, although the CT scan is better at detecting hemorrhage and so is often still chosen for images when intracranial bleeding is a concern.

BONE SCANS

If a bone is not displaced to a sufficient degree for a difference in x-ray absorption, the injury will often not be evident on an x-ray or CT scan. However, at the site of the injury, the bone is very active in trying to repair the damage. A

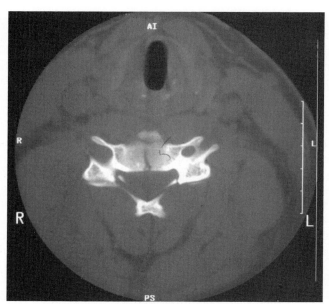

Figure 3-11. ▪ **A CT scan of the fifth cervical vertebrae.** Note the fracture in the midline of the vertebral body.

bone scan can image this activity and thus give evidence of the injury within 24 to 48 hours of the incident, long before other types of imaging would produce any warning signs. The cost of a bone scan is usually about half that of a CT scan.

Bone scans take advantage of the fact that an injured or stressed bone will be actively building more mass or repairing damage by absorbing more calcium and other items from the bloodstream. Blood is drawn from the patient and then "tagged" with a radiopharmaceutical. A radiopharmaceutical is simply a compound that is radioactive, it emits gamma radiation. However, chemically it interacts identically to a nonradioactive pharmaceutical because the number of electrons are the same. Thus the body does not detect any difference. Once the radiopharmaceutical is absorbed in the body at the active site, an external gamma camera can detect where the greatest concentration of radiation is, which is also the site of the most metabolic activity, which is also the site of the injury. Note that these radiopharmaceuticals decay very rapidly and the radiation dose to the patient is minimal.

Figure 3-12 shows a bone scan (Figure 3-12, *A*) and x-ray (Figure 3-12, *B*), respectively, of an injured bone. The bone scan clearly shows an increased uptake on the neck of the left femur, indicating repair is taking place. The x-ray does not indicate any injury at this site.

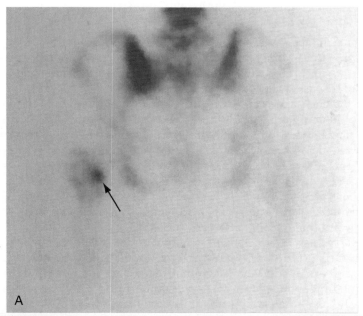

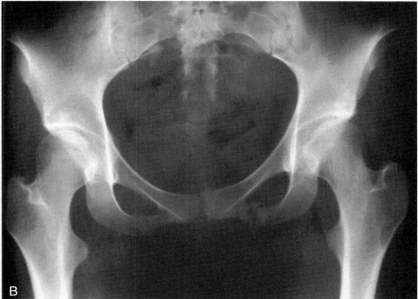

Figure 3-12. ■ Bone scan (A) and x-ray (B) of the femurs. The bone scan **(A)** clearly shows an increased uptake on the neck of the left femur (*arrow*), indicating increased metabolic activity at the site of the injury. **B,** The x-ray does not indicate any injury.

MAGNETIC RESONANCE IMAGING (MRI)
Basic MRI

Magnetic resonance imaging is an amazing tool for the physical therapist—because it gives clear images of soft tissue injuries. It is a relatively recent imaging technique and improvements in its uses are being made every year. This section will discuss the basics.

One of the clear advantages of MRIs is that they involve no radiation dose, unlike the other imaging techniques we have discussed. They require large magnetic fields, but no ionizing radiation is used to create the images.

MRI is a nuclear phenomenon, *not* an atomic phenomenon. It is important to recognize this distinction. Atomic refers to the entire atom (nucleus and orbiting electrons), whereas nuclear refers to the nucleus of the atom. Chemical interactions are atomic; they have to do with the orbiting electrons of different atoms interacting with one another. MRI involves interactions between magnetic fields and the nuclei of atoms.

In simple terms we describe the structure of the atom as a nucleus with neutrons (neutral) and protons (positive) surrounded by orbiting electrons (negative). It is well understood that electrons are not only rotating about the nucleus but also rotating about their own axes, similar to how the earth rotates about the sun—and also rotates daily about its own axis.

Likewise, nucleons (neutrons and protons) spin about their own axes, similar to electron motion, and thus they possess nuclear spin. Nuclear spin is essential to creating an MRI image.

Moving charges create magnetic fields. Since the spinning nucleus has a net positive charge, it creates a dipole magnetic field, shown in Figure 3-13, *A*. The spinning nucleus can be viewed as a microscopic magnet, represented as a

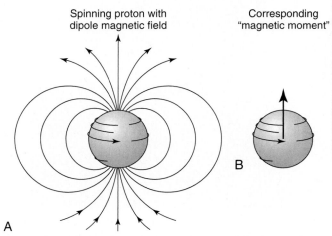

Spinning proton with
dipole magnetic field

Corresponding
"magnetic moment"

B

A

Figure 3-13. ■ **A,** A spinning proton, because it has a net charge and is spinning, creates a magnetic field. **B,** Since this is too elaborate to draw each time, the characteristics of a dipole field are simplified as a single vector, μ, representing the magnetic moment of the dipole field. *(Redrawn from Bushberg JT: The essential physics of medical imaging, ed 2, LWW, Philadelphia, 2002.)*

single vector, μ, shown in Figure 3-13, *B*. The nuclear magnetic moment is the name we give to this vector μ, and it is proportional to the angular momentum of the nucleus. Recall that any object that rotates has an angular momentum.

Moment of inertia is a measure of an object's ability to resist changes in rotational motion. The gyromagnetic ratio (often indicated by the symbol gamma) is the ratio of the nuclear magnetic moment (which measures the angular momentum of the nucleus) to the moment of inertia.

$$\gamma = \frac{\text{nuclear magnetic moment}}{\text{moment of inertia}}$$

The gyromagnetic ratio (gamma) is important because each isotope has a different gamma. This, along with differences in "relaxation times" (which we will discuss shortly) permits the MRI to differentiate between various tissues. Therefore, MRIs can clearly image tears in muscle tissue, and can easily distinguish between tumorous and healthy tissues, and between gray and white matter in the brain.

Many different nuclei could be used for imaging; however, hydrogen is the principal element used in medical imaging with an MRI. It has a large magnetic moment and is abundant in the human body. Hydrogen has a single proton in its nucleus, so the terms *hydrogen*, *proton*, and *nuclei* are often used interchangeably.

Since the spinning nucleus is basically a microscopic magnet, it is affected by an external magnetic field. In MRI a very strong external magnetic field is applied to the body part to be imaged. This causes the millions of nuclei (which are microscopic magnets) to line up either parallel or antiparallel to the external magnetic field (Figure 3-14). A specific radio frequency (RF) pulse is then applied, which inputs energy to the nuclei and causes them to be "tipped" from their orientation. When the RF pulse is turned off, the nuclei realign, and in doing so emit an RF pulse. The duration, location, and strength of that returning RF pulse is collected, interpreted, and processed to create an image of the site.

If equal numbers of nuclei lined up parallel and antiparallel, there would be no net magnetization caused by these nuclei because they would cancel each other out.

However, this doesn't happen. There is a very small difference between the number that line up parallel and antiparallel. If a million protons are immersed in a strong external magnetic field, about three more protons would be in the parallel state (lower energy) than in the antiparallel state. This sounds like a ridiculously small amount. However, consider that in a cubic millimeter of tissue there are approximately 10^{19} protons. Therefore, there are approximately 3×10^{13} more protons in the parallel state than in the antiparallel state. This is more than sufficient to produce an MRI signal. The nuclei lining up parallel and antiparallel are often referred to as being in spin-up and spin-down states, respectively.

Since there are unequal numbers of protons in the spin-up and spin-down states, they don't all cancel each other out, and there is a net magnetization along the direction of the applied external magnetic field as a result of the millions of nuclei. This is illustrated in Figure 3-15 where M_0 represents the net magnetization vector.

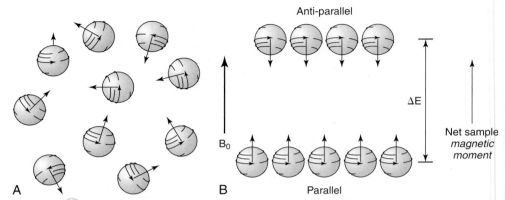

Figure 3-14. ■ **Representation of the magnetic moments (μ) of protons with and without an external magnetic field. A,** In the absence of any strong external magnetic field, a group of protons all have random orientations of their nuclear magnetic moments, μ, and thus the net magnetic moment of the sample is zero. **B,** When an external magnetic field (B_0) is applied, the orientation is no longer random, the protons align with their nuclear magnetic moments, μ, parallel or antiparallel to the field. There is a slight preference for alignment parallel, which is at a lower energy state. Thus a net magnetic moment of the sample exists in the direction of B_0, as shown by the arrow at the far right in the figure. *(Redrawn from Bushberg JT: The essential physics of medical imaging, ed 2, LWW, Philadelphia, 2002.)*

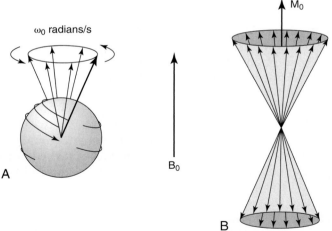

Figure 3-15. ■ **A,** Under the influence of an external magnetic field, B_0 each proton precesses about the direction of B_0. **B,** In any object there are many million of protons precessing, the net effect (because of the excess protons aligned parallel to B_0) is a net magnetization (M_0) in the direction of B_0. There is no magnetization in the perpendicular direction because there is no preferred direction other than the z-direction when precessing. *(Redrawn from Bushberg JT: The essential physics of medical imaging, ed 2, LWW, Philadelphia, 2002.)*

It is interesting to note that the number of excess protons is a function of the magnitude of the external magnetic field (as well as the temperature, which stays fairly constant in a body). This accounts for the increasing strength of the magnetic field in each generation of MRI machines.

As illustrated in Figure 3-15, the protons in the spin-up and spin-down states are not just aligned about the z-axis (the direction of the large external magnetic field), but are also precessing about this axis. This precession is due to the torque caused by the interaction of the external magnetic field and the nuclear magnetic moment. This is similar to the torque a spinning top feels due to the force of gravity, which causes it to precess. If a top is not spinning, the gravitational force simply causes it to fall over. However, if a top is spinning, the interaction of the spinning and the gravitation force create a torque, which cause it to precess rather than fall (Figure 3-16).

In our case, a torque is felt by the spinning nuclei because of the magnetic field, rather than the gravitational field. By convention, the z-direction is the direction of the strong external magnetic field. Since the proton is positively charged, the direction of the magnetic moment vector, μ, and the angular momentum vector, L, are identical. As can be seen in Figure 3-17, the direction of the torque is perpendicular to both the magnetic field B_0 and the angular

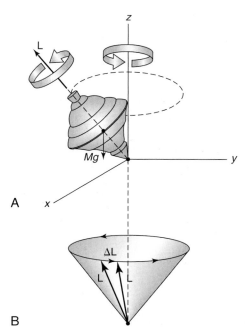

■ **Figure 3-16.** ■ **Precessional motion of a top spinning about its symmetric axis. A,** The gravitational force creates a torque in the x-y plane. **B,** Since the change in angular momentum, dL/dt is also equal to the torque; this implies the change in angular momentum is perpendicular to L, causing a precession about the z-axis.

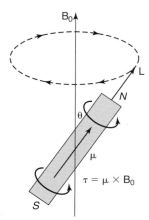

$$B_0$$
$$L$$
$$N$$
$$\theta$$
$$\mu$$
$$\tau = \mu \times B_0$$
$$S$$

Figure 3-17. ■ A spinning nucleus can be represented as a spinning bar magnet. The direction of the vectors representing the nuclear magnetic moment, μ, and the angular momentum, L, are identical. When placed in an external magnetic field, B_0, the spinning nucleus experiences a torque equal to μ × B_0, which causes it to precess about the z-axis. (By convention the z-axis is defined as the direction of the external magnetic field B_0.) This is similar to the torque (r × Mg) felt by a spinning top in a gravitational field (see Figure 3-16).

momentum $\left(\tau = \mu \times B_o = \dfrac{dL}{dt} \right)$, creating a change in angular momentum that causes the proton to precess about the z-axis.

If we examine a single proton or nucleus precessing about the z-axis, we would see a component of magnetization along the direction of the external magnetic field (z-direction) and a component along the plane perpendicular to that (x-y plane). However when we examine millions of nuclei, which are randomly distributed, the net effect is a magnetization in the z-direction, because the magnetizations in the xy plane cancel each other out (see Figure 3-15 B). The result of this precession is still a net magnetization in the direction of the applied magnetic field, the z-axis.

Larmor Frequency

If the net magnetization (M_0) remains parallel to the external applied magnetic field (B_0), it is difficult to measure because it is masked by the large external field ($M_0 <<< B_0$). When the RF pulse is applied, the net magnetization vector is now at some angle (the angle depends on the duration of the RF pulse) at which it precesses about the original direction.

A very important concept in MRI is the Larmor frequency. The Larmor frequency (ω) is equal to the product of the gyromagnetic ratio (γ) and the magnitude of the external magnetic field (B_0). Since the Larmor frequency depends on

Table 3-1
Spin, Gyromagnetic Ratios, and the Natural Abundance of Selected Nuclides*

Nucleus	Spin	Gyromagnetic ratio $10^7 T^{-1}s^{-1}$	Natural Abundance (%)
1 H	½	26.75	99.985
2 H	1	4.11	0.015
13 C	½	6.73	1.108
19 F	½	25.18	100.00
14 N	1	1.93	99.63
31 P	½	10.84	100.0

*T stands for Tesla (1 Tesla = 10^4 Gauss. The earth's magnetic field is around 0.5 Gauss.)
Adapted from http://web.mit.edu/5.311/www/NMR.pdf

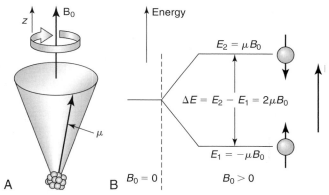

Figure 3-18. ■ **A,** When a nucleus is placed in an external magnetic field, B_0, the magnetic moment precesses about the magnetic field with a frequency proportional to the field. **B,** When placed in an external magnetic field a proton can occupy one of two energy states. When the spin is aligned with the field, this is the lower energy state E_1 (spin-up state), and the higher energy state E_2 corresponds to the case where the spin is opposite the field (spin-down state). The energy difference between the two states is proportional to the external magnetic field B_0. *(Redrawn from Bushberg JT: The essential physics of medical imaging, ed 2, LWW, Philadelphia, 2002.)*

γ and different isotopes have different γ (as shown in Table 3-1), then the Larmor frequency is isotope specific (in almost all medical imaging this isotope is hydrogen).

$$\bar{\omega} = \gamma\, B_0$$

From Figure 3-18 one can see that the energy difference between the spin-up and spin-down states varies with the strength of the external magnetic field.

If a stronger magnetic field is applied, the energy difference between the two spin states increases. Since the Larmor frequency is also related to the external magnetic field we can obtain a relationship between the Larmor frequency (ω) and the energy difference.

$\Delta E = \omega \hbar$ (where $\hbar$ is Planck's constant divided by 2π)

To get an image, the applied RF pulse mentioned above must be at this exact Larmor frequency. Since the Larmor frequency is related to the energy difference (ΔE) between the spin-up and spin-down states, the system can only absorb the energy from the RF pulse if it is at this exact frequency. This has to do with quantum physics. The energy difference between the spin-up and spin-down states is quantized. A good analogy is the difference between stairs and a ramp. Walking up a ramp, you can take any step length you want; walking up stairs, you can only take specific step lengths, so the size of your steps is quantized. If you take a smaller step than the height of the step, you won't progress up the stairs. Likewise if ΔE is not equal to the energy difference between the states, the energy won't be absorbed.

When the energy from the RF pulse is absorbed, it can cause nuclei to go from the spin-up state to the spin-down state. The duration and amplitude of the RF pulses determine how many protons absorb the energy and "flip" from one energy state to the other. Once the RF pulse is stopped, the nuclei return to their original configuration, emitting energy equal to the energy difference (ΔE) between the two spin states. It is the analysis of this emitted energy (in the form of an RF pulse), and the relaxation times (we are about to get to that), that allows such phenomenal images to be created with an MRI.

Since the Larmor frequency depends on the gyromagnetic ratio, and a signal can only be achieved if the RF pulse is applied at the Larmor frequency, the gyromagnetic ratio (γ) is important. As PTs you do not need to know the values of the gyromagnetic ratio (γ) or the Larmor frequency. This is a matter for the MRI technician who runs the machine and creates the image. It is the specificity of the Larmor frequency that allows a particular plane in the patient to be imaged, which will become clear once we discuss magnetic field gradients.

Flips

A term seen frequently in discussing MRI is 90° and 180° flip. When an external magnetic field is applied, all the microscopic magnets (the nuclei) line up so they are precessing either parallel or antiparallel (spin-up or spin-down). Recall that the vector representing the net magnetization is either parallel or antiparallel. This net magnetization is much smaller than the applied magnetic field. Therefore to measure the net magnetization, an RF pulse is applied, the net effect of which is to "flip" the direction of the net magnetization. The longer the time the RF pulse is applied, the greater the angle. (The most common angles are 90° and 180°.) When the RF pulse is turned off, the computer measures the time it takes for the net magnetization vector to return to the direction of the applied external magnetic field. This time is affected by the environment of the nuclei, which translates into images of the environment (such as muscles, tissues, etc.).

T1 and T2

Creating an image requires contrast between shades of black and white, and the contrast in an MRI image comes from properties known as T1 (spin-lattice relaxation time, longitudinal relaxation time, or thermal relaxation time), and T2 (spin-spin relaxation time). As will be shown, T1 and T2 images complement one another.

Images in MRI are usually identified as T1 or T2 images. T1 and T2 are biologically significant characteristics of the body; they are inherent parameters of the tissues. Here is where the power of MRI is evident. X-ray images achieve contrast because of differences in how much of the x-rays are absorbed by different organs, tissues, or structures in the patient's body. Especially in soft tissue injury, there is not much difference in the absorption of x-rays. However, there is a significant difference in T1, T2, and other measurements made in MRI between injured and healthy tissues.

T1 measures the spin-lattice interactions, which are affected by the dissipation of absorbed energy into the surrounding molecular lattice. T1 is related to the time it takes (after say a 90° pulse) the longitudinal magnetization, M_z, to return to its original value, M_0. When an RF pulse is applied and the net magnetization is flipped from the z-direction into the x-y plane, it gradually returns to its original orientation once the RF pulse is stopped. This recovery time is actually an exponential function (Figure 3-19).

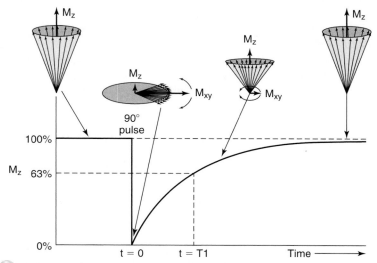

Figure 3-19. ■ After a 90° pulse, the net magnetization is now in the x-y plane (M_{xy}), and the longitudinal magnetization (M_z) is zero. When the pulse is turned off, the magnetization exponentially returns to the original, z, orientation. T1 represents the time at which 63% of the original magnetization in the z-direction is recovered. *(Redrawn from Bushberg JT: The essential physics of medical imaging, ed 2, LWW, Philadelphia, 2002.)*

T1 is the time it takes to recover 63% of its original value. T1 times are longer the greater the water content—so they are longest (~3 sec) in pure water and cerebrospinal fluid (CSF), shorter in tissues with significant water content such as gray matter in the brain, and shortest in fat tissue (a few hundred milliseconds).

Figure 3-20 shows a T1 weighted image of the brain and spinal column. One can clearly see the spinal cord. Note the cerebrospinal fluid is the dark edge around the cord. The bodies of the cervical vertebrae are also clearly evident.

Since the spinning nuclei are microscopic magnets, they are affected by surrounding magnetic fields. This includes not only the strong external magnetic field applied, but also the micromagnetic fields created by the surrounding nuclei (which can all be considered minimagnets as they have a positive charge and are spinning). T2 measures these spin-spin interactions. In other words, T2 is affected by the interaction, due to the magnetic fields, between a particular nuclei and surrounding nuclei. After an RF pulse is applied, T2 decay measures the time for the transverse magnetization to decay to 37% of the original value (Figure 3-21). The T2 decay measures the degree to which the nuclei become out of phase with one another.

It's as if you had a bunch of marching teenagers initially listening to the marching band (the external magnetic field). If they each then started to listen to their own music (the magnetic fields they each create) this would influence them and probably those right next to them. When they started off together they would all be "in phase" with one another, but as they progressed they would be influenced by their 'local' surroundings (their own music and that of the ones right next to them) and get out of step.

Immediately after the RF pulse is applied, the millions of hydrogen nuclei are in phase with one another. However, the transverse magnetization decreases because the local magnetic fields vary for each nuclei because of the type of nuclei in close proximity, thus changing the phase of the precessing nuclei. $T2^*$ is another term you will sometimes see on MRIs. $T2^*$ is always shorter than T2. It is a measure of the exponential decay due to both intrinsic and extrinsic magnetic field variations, T2 only measures relative to the intrinsic magnetic properties. Figure 3-22 shows a T2 weighted image.

T2 values are always less than T1 values. T2 values are shortest in soft tissues (50 to 100 msec) and longer in fluids (several hundred milliseconds). **Diseased tissues typically have higher water content than healthy tissues.** This leads to a difference (and thus a contrast in the image) between the T1 and T2 values of the normal healthy tissues and those of diseased tissues (the diseased tissues typically having longer T1 and T2 values). This is why, on T2 images, diseased tissues typically show up as white and bright. Table 3-2 shows some typical T1 and T2 times for different tissues in the brain.

Figure 3-23 shows a third type of weighting called inversion recovery (IR). Although T1 and T2 weighted images are the most common, many others are in use, allowing differing degrees of contrast.

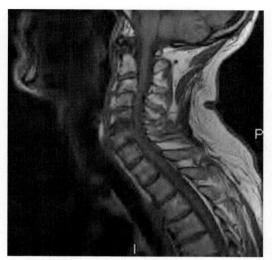

Figure 3-20. ■ MRI image, which is T1 weighted, of the spinal cord and cervical vertebrae.

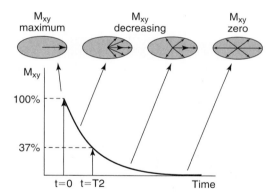

Figure 3-21. ■ After a 90° pulse, the net magnetization is now in the x-y plane and has phase coherence. However, due mainly to interactions with the magnetic fields of other nuclei, the many nuclei become out of phase with one another. This occurs exponentially. T2 is the time over which the signal decays to 37% of the maximum transverse magnetization. T2 is always shorter than T1. *(Redrawn from Bushberg JT: The essential physics of medical imaging, ed 2, LWW, Philadelphia, 2002.)*

Spin-Echo Pulse Sequence

One of the most commonly used pulse sequences in clinical MR imaging is the spin-echo pulse sequence. This begins with a 90° pulse, which tips the net magnetization into the transverse plane. This is followed at a later time (TE/2) by a 180° pulse, which eliminates the effects of the magnetic field inhomogenities.

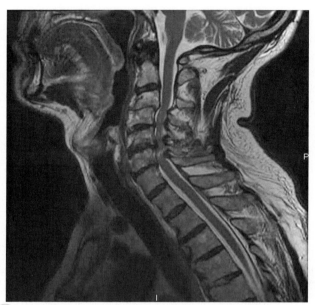

Figure **3-22.** ■ MRI image showing T2 weighted image.

Table 3-2
Examples of T_1 and T_2 Values of Different Tissues in the Brain

Tissue Type	T_1 (ms)	T_2 (ms)
White matter	871	87
Gray matter	515	74
Cerebrospinal fluid	1900	250

From: http://www.es.oersted.dtu.dk/~masc/T1_T2.htm

At a time of TE/2 further along, the signal echo (or spin echo) is obtained. Thus TE stands for "time of echo," as the signal echo occurs at TE after the 90° pulse. Sometime later this entire sequence is repeated. The repetition time (TR) is the time between consecutive 90° pulses.

It is important to note that T1 and T2 are inherent tissue parameters. The goal of medical imaging is to translate these inherent differences between tissues into an image contrast. To do that, the technician can select different pulse sequences, different TE, different TR, different angles, etc. When you examine an MRI it will typically indicate what the TE, TR, etc. values were. This aids in interpreting the image.

A T1 weighted image, see Figure 3-20, (relatively short TR and short TE) will have bright areas indicating short T1 values (such as fat) and dark areas with

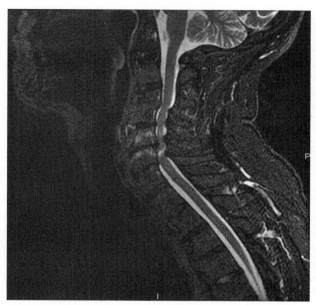

Figure 3-23. ■ MRI image using inversion recovery (IR) of the spinal cord and cervical vertebrae.

tissues having long T1 values (such as cerebrospinal fluid). A short TR (relative to T1 values) will mean that the longitudinal magnetization is only partially recovered in each sequence. For a given TR, a tissue with a shorter T1 (such as fat) will recover more of the longitudinal magnetization, and show up as bright. A tissue with a lot of water in it (such as cerebrospinal fluid or a lesion), which has a longer T1, will not have enough time to recover nearly as much of the longitudinal magnetization, so it will appear dark. If TR is long, there is little T1 weighting because all the longitudinal magnetization is fully recovered, and there is little contrast between tissues with varying T1 values.

On the other hand, TE controls the amount of T2 weighting in an image, see Figure 3-23. If TE is long compared with the T2 values of the tissues of interest, this gives enough time for the transverse dephasing to occur. Tissues with varying dephasing (different T2) will be emphasized. A T2 weighted image has a longer TR—so that there is little T1 weighting and longer TE—so that there is more time for transverse dephasing. Note that similar to a long TR with a T1 weighted image, if TE is made too long, signals from all the tissues will be similar and little contrast will result. If TE is made too short, little transverse dephasing will occur, and T2 differences will not be apparent. A T2 weighted image inverts the tissue contrast seen in T1 weighted image (so that fat is darker than CSF instead of brighter).

Figure 3-24 summarizes some of these differences and demonstrates the complementary nature of T1 and T2 weighted images. This shows a gradient of

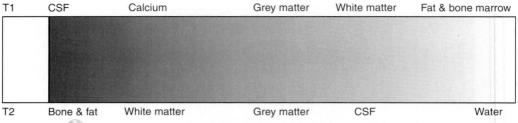

Figure 3-24. ■ This black to white gradient summarizes the contrast differences for T1 and T2 weighted images.

black to white. In a T2 weighted image bone and fat are dark and tissues with high water content are white. In a T1 weighted image the opposite is true.

It is essential to recognize that almost every MR image is actually a "mixed" image. For example, not all the contrast in a T2 weighted image is due to differences in T2. Since organs and tissues have various values for T1 and T2 tissues in different parts of the image may have different weighting.

Gradients

Another very important advantage of MRI is the ability to create tomographic images of any orientation (axial, coronals, and sagittal). This creation of tomographic images (or slices) is obtained using magnetic field gradients. By changing the magnetic field in a linear fashion across the patient's body (in any plane), and then changing the RF pulse correspondingly, a specific location can be targeted. The slight change in the magnetic field is done with gradient coils. There are separate gradient coils in each plane (x, y, and z).

It is important not to confuse the direction of the gradient and the direction of the magnetic field. The external magnetic field is always in the same direction (by convention this is designated the z-direction). The gradient coils produce *changes* in the magnetic field in a specific direction. For example, the y-gradient coils produce a variation (a gradient) in the magnitude of the magnetic field in the y-direction. This is perhaps easiest to understand with a specific example.

Let's examine an MRI of the head. Assume the patient is placed in the MRI machine lying face up, so that the z-direction, which is the direction the external magnetic field is applied, goes from toes to head. We will let the x-direction be horizontal, going from ear to ear, and the y-direction be vertical, going from the back of the head to the face (Figure 3-25).

Let's apply gradients in the y-direction. In other words, the external magnetic field, B, which is in the z-direction, varies in strength in the y-direction, with the strongest B field being at the back of the head and the smallest being in the plane of the face. This is shown as arrows superimposed on the head in the image on the right.

The Larmor frequency, ω, depends on the external magnetic field ($\omega = \gamma B$). Due to the gradients, each horizontal plane shown will respond to a slightly

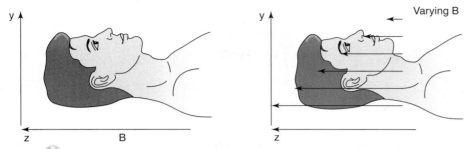

Figure 3-25. ■ The external magnetic field is in the z-direction and the gradients are in the y-direction. To create a tomographic image, a particular Larmor frequency, corresponding to a specific value of the B field is chosen.

different Larmor frequency. The energy difference between the spin-up and spin-down states is also a function of the magnetic field, and therefore related to the Larmor frequency. Since the energy is quantized, only RF pulses applied at the Larmor frequency can be absorbed by the nuclei and create an image.

To obtain an image of a particular plane in the y-direction, let's say at the ear level, the RF pulse is tuned so that it is at the Larmor frequency corresponding to the B field in this specific plane. Thus only the nuclei with that particular magnetic field applied to them will absorb the energy and cause the nuclei in that plane to flip from spin-up to spin-down. When the RF pulse is turned off, these nuclei return to their original orientation (as discussed earlier), emitting an RF pulse that can be detected (and T1, T2, etc., determined), thus creating an image of that plane. Nuclei in planes above or below that level will not respond to the RF pulse because the energy is not exactly at the right value to be absorbed.

To obtain an image of a plane closer to the front of the face, a slightly shorter Larmor frequency would be selected, relating to the slightly smaller B field applied to that plane.

If the gradients were applied in the x-direction (Figure 3-26) then the external magnetic field (which is still in the z-direction) would vary in strength from one ear to the other. To image a particular slice, the specific Larmor frequency associated with the B field in that slice would be selected, and only nuclei in that particular B field would absorb the energy, resulting in an image. Likewise a plane could be selected in the axial direction when the gradients are applied in the z-direction.

One of the real advantages of an MRI is that gradients can be applied in either the x-, y- or z- direction, thus allowing axial, coronals, and sagittal images to be obtained.

Comparison of Various Imaging Modalities

Many people confuse CT scans and MRIs because the equipment is similar in appearance (a gantry sliding the patient into a cavernlike hole, lots of computers, etc.) and both produce tomographic images. A key difference is that x-ray

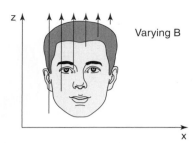

Figure 3-26. ■ The external magnetic field is in the z-direction and the gradients are in the x-direction, from ear to ear. Thus a tomographic slice in the x-direction can be selected by choosing a specific Larmor frequency corresponding to the B field at a particular location across the patient's head.

attenuation determines CT images; in other words, the types and amounts of elements present and their effective atomic number. In contrast, MRI signals are strongly influenced by chemical interactions, molecular motions, and fluid flow. Another important difference is MRIs do not expose the patient to radiation doses.

Although the spatial resolution is not as good for MRIs as it is for CT images, the contrast resolution is very much better. This is also true when comparing CT scans with radiological images, CT scans have much better contrast resolution than radiological images (at the cost of higher radiation doses to the patient).

MRIs will never replace CT scans; they are both important imaging tools. However, MRIs are far superior for soft tissue injury. Another important distinction is that CT scans are often used in emergency situations, whereas MRIs require more time to take and are more often used in follow-up or nonemergency situations. Almost all hospitals have CT scanners, but especially in remote locations, MRIs are not as easily available. MRIs are also much more expensive.

It is important to recognize that, although MRIs and CTs are tomographic images, "simple" x-rays are valuable in many situations, especially when looking at anatomical structures. As you progress through the different chapters you will discover many valuable x-ray images.

We also briefly discussed bone scans, which image physiologic changes because of injury, and give therapists and doctors an insight not gained by the other imaging techniques.

There are many other imaging techniques not covered in this book. Many of the most recent advances in health care have been because of better imaging techniques.

REFERENCES

1. *http://www.sprawls.org/resources/DIGRAD/module.htm#18*
2. Bushberg JT: The essential physics of medical imaging, ed 2, LWW. Philadelphia, 2002.

4 The Cervical Spine

INTRODUCTION ▄▄▄▄▄

Remarks

The cervical spine is best analyzed on plain-routine films as three distinct anatomical regions: the first cervical segment (C1), the second cervical segment (C2), and the remainder of the distal cervical segments. In one study, a series of standard-routine x-rays of the cervical spine has been shown to be 84% accurate in detecting fractures of the cervical spine.[1]

C1 is unique for several reasons, and these place it at risk for pathologic conditions that are not normally encountered at the subsequent vertebral segments. C1 has no vertebral body, which means it has no annulus for stabilization. It is wrapped around the cephalad projection of the vertebral body of the C2 that is known as the "odontoid" or "dens," not unlike a ring around a post. C1 is held in proper alignment with the odontoid by several ligaments, the most important being the transverse ligament. It is dependent upon the integrity of the transverse ligament for its alignment. The transverse ligament is the primary restraint that prevents anterior displacement of C1 on C2.[2,3,4] The articular facets at this spinal level, unlike those at lower levels, are more horizontally oriented in the anteroposterior (AP) plane to facilitate rotation, but they offer little bony resistance to anterior displacement.

Ligamentous incompetence can be due to congenital laxity, as is sometimes found accompanying Down syndrome. The rupture of the transverse ligament by trauma or progressive disease processes (rheumatoid arthritis [RA]) may result in an unstable C1 segment and may put the upper cervical cord at risk. C1 is unique because it lacks an intervertebral disk and the shock absorption that the combination of the nucleus pulposus and the elasticity of the annulus provide and the stabilization that a proximal and distal annulus would provide. The absence of a disk places this segment at particular risk from trauma when the axial cervical spine is loaded. Examples of this axial loading may occur in diving, football, rugby tackles and the rugby "scrum," wrestling, motor vehicle accidents, trampolines, etc. The articular facets of C1, although horizontal in the AP plane, are wedge shaped in a lateral to medial plane with the medial dimension smaller than the lateral dimension (Figures 4-1 and 4-2).

Note the acute angle in this view of a fracture of C1 at *both* the facets of C1 and the articulation of C1 with the occiput at the base of the skull. An axial load applied through the skull to the wedge-

shaped articular facets of C1, the occiput, and C2 causes the ring-shaped C1 to be forced laterally and often results in fractures of the ring. This is known as a "Jefferson's fracture" and is evidenced on the odontoid or "open-mouth" view of C1 as lateral displacement of the articular facets and/or lateral masses. This displacement can be unilateral or bilateral. During this traumatic process, the transverse ligament can be torn or avulsed (Figure 4-3).

A fracture of the C1 ring with the lateral masses laterally but equally displaced on the superior facets of C2 is shown in Figure 4-4. A unilateral fracture or avulsion of the transverse ligament of C1 is shown in Figure 4-2. This fracture demonstrates the paradox of one side of the avulsion fragment that moves

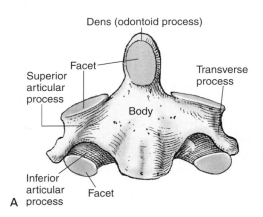

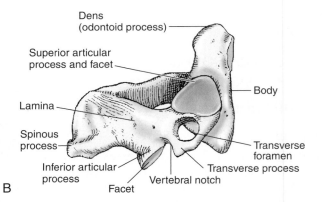

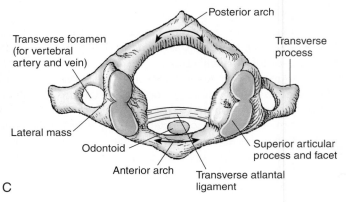

Figure 4-1. ■ **Depicts the relationship of the C1 ring around the odontoid of C2.** Note the wedged shape of C1 lateral masses in the AP view (A). This suggests that an axial load could drive the C1 ring laterally. The lateral view (B) depicts the separation of the anterior odontoid from the C1 right. The distance between the two is the ADI, which should not exceed 3 mm (C). (*From Frank ED: Merrill's atlas of radiographic positioning and procedures, 3 volume set, ed 11, St. Louis, Mosby, 2007.*)

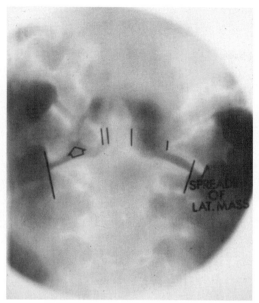

F*igure* 4-2. ■ This open-mouth view demonstrates several problems. Note that the C1 right lateral mass overhangs the C2 facet. Although the left lateral mass is displaced laterally, there is a bone fragment between the lateral mass and the odontoid process.

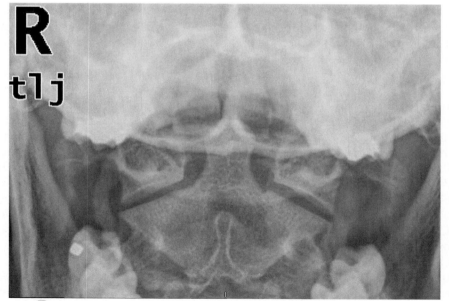

F*igure* 4-3. ■ Represents a normal odontoid view. The lateral masses are aligned with the C2 facets. The odontoid process is centered on the C1 ring, and there are no lucencies in the odontoid process.

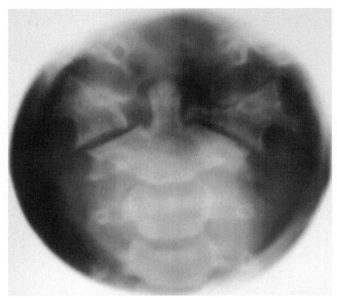

Figure 4-4. ■ Although the space between the lateral masses and the odontoid appear to be equal in this view, note that the lateral masses overhang the C2 facets on both sides, demonstrating a burst fracture of C1.

medially because the transverse ligament is still attached, while the remainder of the same side's lateral mass remains in alignment with the lateral mass below. The facet on the opposite side moves laterally to overhang the facet below.

The fractures or instabilities that may not show up on plain films or those that require more thorough evaluation are imaged with CT or MRI for definitive diagnosis, as shown in Figure 4-5. This figure shows a lateral film that demonstrates a fracture in the vertebral body of C5 and stabilization at that level and "tongs" for traction on the skull. A CT scan of multiple fractures of C5 as a result of a motorcycle accident that more clearly delineates the extent of the fractures is shown in Figure 4-6.

C2 is unique because the proximal portion of its vertebral body projects cephalad through the ring of C1 as a solid bony projection into and through the ring of C1 and serves as an anchor and/or faux vertebral body for C1 (see Figure 4-3). Whereas this arrangement facilitates excellent rotational movement at this segment, it also results in an inherently unstable segment. This projection of the vertebral body of C2 cephalad through another vertebral segment is unique among the vertebrae. The odontoid is the "pillar" around which the ring of C1 rotates and to which C1 is anchored by the transverse ligament. C2 has no intervertebral disk between it and C1 since the odontoid is a solid projection of bone. The odontoid, or dens, can be fractured by trauma, a developmental congenital malformation, or failure to fuse. The fractures of the odontoid are categorized as: types I, II, and III based upon the location and direction of the fracture, as shown in Figure 4-7.[5,6]

Type I is an oblique fracture through the upper one third of the odontoid and is relatively rare.[6]

Type II is a transverse fracture through the base of the odontoid where it joins and is contiguous with the normal body of C2.

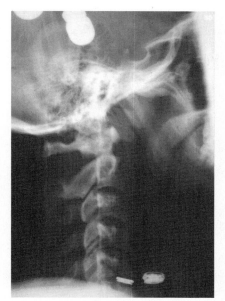

Figure 4-5. ■ **Lateral view of the cervical spine.** The height of the anterior C5 vertebral body is less than the other vertebrae, suggesting a compression fracture. The metal objects seen in the skull are tongs for traction and stabilization of the fracture. (See Figure 4-6; a CT scan of the C5, clearly demonstrating the fracture.)

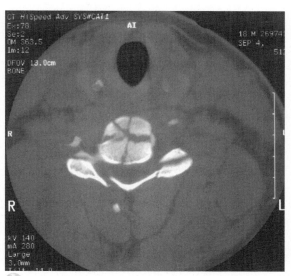

Figure 4-6. ■ **A CT scan of the C5 vertebral body of an individual involved in a motorcycle accident.** The C5 body is clearly shown to be broken into five pie-shaped wedges.

Stability is often compromised in this type of dens fracture.

Type III is a fracture of the odontoid down into the body of C2. These have a component of neurologic compromise in 5% to 10% of the injuries.[6]

Figure 4-8 depicts a type III odontoid fracture portion: Note the normal alignment of the lateral masses to the odontoid and the superior articular facets of C2 below and that there is no lateral overhang of the facets of C1 relative to C2.

The remainder of the cervical vertebrae—C3 through C7—are similar to one another relative to size, components, shape, density, and dimensions and can be compared with reasonable accuracy to the segments above and below.

The spine is divided into three columns from anterior to posterior based upon a study performed by Denis.[7] This concept supplanted the prior "two-column spine" concept because Denis demonstrated that the majority of spinal fractures are in the anterior half of the vertebral bodies of the lower thoracolumbar spine and are flexion-compression fractures. He proposed that the three-column spine be divided into the following sections: The first is the anterior half of the vertebral body, the second is the posterior half of the vertebral body and the pedicles, and the third section of the three-column spine is from the pedicles to the rear of the spinous processes. The majority of the fractures in Denis's study were in column 1 at the L1 level. Allen modified the Denis classification to be applicable to the lower cervical spine.[8]

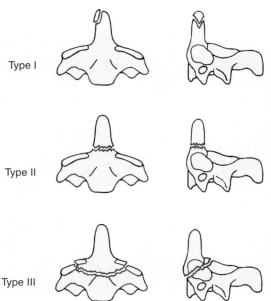

Type I

Type II

Type III

***Figure* 4-7.** ■ **Demonstrates a classification system for labeling different types of odontoid fractures.** *Type I* fractures are stable because the odontoid prevents shifting of the C1 ring. *Type II* fractures are unstable, having lost the bony stability of the odontoid. *Type III* fracture through the body of C2. *(From Browner BD et al: Skeletal trauma: Basic science, management, and reconstruction, ed 3, Philadelphia, 2003, Saunders.)*

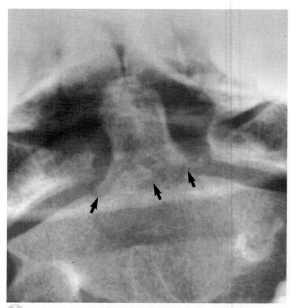

***Figure* 4-8.** ■ **Demonstrates a type III fracture in the spongy bone at the base of the odontoid.** *(From Browner BD et al:* Skeletal trauma: Basic science, management, and reconstruction, *ed 3, Philadelphia, 2003, Saunders.)*

OBJECTIVES

1. Recall the five standard cervical spine views and their purposes.
2. Identify normal and abnormal alignment of the five standard views.
3. Identify normal and abnormal densities or dimensions of the cervical spine.
4. Identify normal and abnormal cartilage.
5. Identify normal and abnormal soft tissue findings in the cervical spine.
6. Identify film abnormalities, given a history and x-ray film.
7. Use information from x-ray films to adjust a physical therapy treatment program.

STANDARD VIEWS

There are five separate views required to perform the basic evaluation of the cervical spine with plain film x-rays:
1. Odontoid (open-mouth) view
2. AP
3. Left oblique
4. Right oblique
5. Lateral

EVALUATION OF THE CERVICAL SPINE USING ABCS
Odontoid (Open-Mouth) View

The odontoid view is an AP view taken with the patient supine and his or her mouth open. The beam is directed into the open mouth toward the pharynx, and the film is placed between the posterior portion of the patient's cervical spine and occiput and the table (Figures 4-9 and 4-10).

   Alignment

   This unique view is designed to demonstrate the odontoid and lateral masses of C1. In regular AP exposure, C1 would be obscured by the mandible and the dentition. The alignment points on this view are: the distance

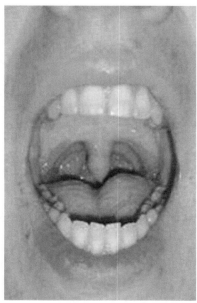

Figure **4-9.** ■ Demonstrates the patient's position necessary to take the open-mouth or odontoid view.

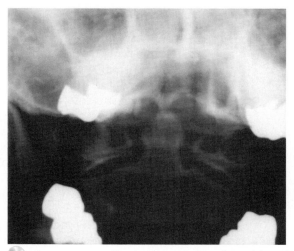

Figure **4-10.** ■ Demonstrates the odontoid and lateral masses of C1 seen in an odontoid view. Alignment and bony density are normal.

between the lateral edges of the odontoid and the medial edges of the lateral masses (articular facets) are symmetrical. The inferior surface of the articular facets of C1 must not be displaced laterally over the lateral portion of the superior articular facets of C2. These articular surfaces of C1 and C2 should be parallel. Figure 4-3 is a normal view with lateral masses labeled to show: (1) no lateral overhang, (2) equidistance from lateral borders of the odontoid to the medial borders of the lateral masses, and (3) parallel distance between the inferior margins of the facets of C1 and the superior margins of the facets of C2.

Figure 4-4 demonstrates a fracture of C1 and equal lateral displacements of the lateral masses of C1.

Bone Density and Dimension
The odontoid should have no lucencies in the proximal portion, base, or into the vertebral body of the second cervical vertebra (see Figure 4-8). The bones of the odontoid and C1 should be of equal, consistent density with no unexplained lucencies through the bones.

Cartilage
Since C1 has no intervertebral disk, the cartilage portion of the open-mouth view is focused on the articular surfaces of the facets to ensure they are parallel and equally spaced with no bone on bone surfaces.

Soft Tissue
The open-mouth view of C1 reveals very little in the way of information about the surrounding soft tissue.

AP View

The AP view is taken with the patient supine or sitting. This view is to assess the anteroposterior portion of the cervical spine from C3 to C7.

Alignment
A vertical line is drawn superior to inferior along the spinous processes to assess any segmental rotation that is evident from this projection. Remember that cervical spinous processes are bifid (i.e., they split posteriorly into two small projections). The pedicles are identified at each segment and assessed for indications of segmental rotation. A vertical assessment of the lateral borders of the vertebral bodies of this view is performed to assess any segmental lateral displacement or unilateral segmental "tilting." The uncinate joints (two at each superior and inferior portion of the vertebral bodies) are evaluated for osteophytes or degenerative changes. Figures 4-11 and 4-12 are examples of normal AP views of the cervical spine (Figures 4-11 and 4-12).

Bone Density and Dimension
The individual pedicles and vertebral bodies are assessed for any changes in density or dimensions. Segments above and below are used for comparison and if necessary measure the horizontal and vertical dimensions in millimeters for comparison.

Cartilage
The assessment of cartilage is best evaluated on the lateral cervical views.

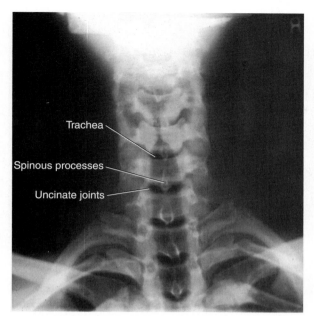

Figure 4-11. ■ **AP view of a normal cervical spine.** The spinous processes are aligned. Bone density is consistent from level to level. Cartilage space is not well defined in this view. Note the dark central area in the midline. This is the air-filled trachea. In some trauma and disease processes, the trachea may be displaced to the side.

Soft Tissue

This view is extremely valuable for evaluating the alignment of the vertical, dark, shadowlike (decreased density) trachea that should be seen midline within the vertebrae from the larynx inferior to the base of the cervical spine. If the trachea is not midline, it may indicate the presence of: a tumor (Pancoast's tumor), a pneumothorax, or hemothorax (Figure 4-13). In Figure 4-13, note that a Pancoast's tumor has displaced the trachea toward the right as we view this film and destroyed the first rib.

Left and Right Oblique Views

There are always two oblique views taken both in the cervical spine and the lumbar spine, and these should be compared for side-to-side consistency. They are primarily to evaluate the status of the intervertebral foramina in the cervical spine, but also provide excellent views of the pedicles and the articular facets. The dimensions of the foramina above and those below are good measures of the appropriate patency of each opening, the existence of osteophytes, or stenotic changes. It is critical to correlate any x-ray changes with the patient's symptoms and examination and to evaluate the existence of progression for any of the changes in the foramen. A progressive weakness in the appropriate myotome, a

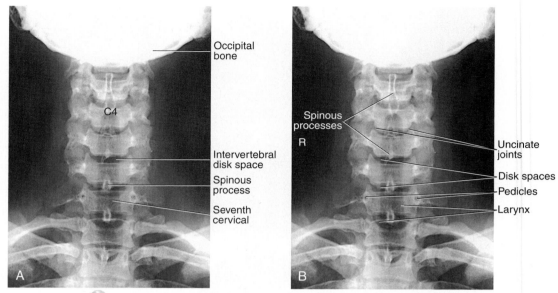

Figure **4-12** **A** and **B,** Alignment points along the spinous process. *(From Frank ED:* Merrill's atlas of radiographic positioning and procedures, *ed 11, St. Louis, Mosby 2007.)*

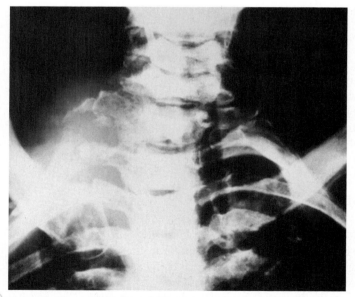

Figure **4-13.** ■ **Note the white mass on the left side of this film in the upper lung area.** This is a Pancoast's tumor. Also note that the dark trachea has been displaced from midline to the right side by the growing mass of the tumor.

diminished reflex, or increasing radicular pain may indicate the existence of a tumor (such as a schwannoma), progressive stenosis caused by a progressive nuclear herniation, or bony growth as a result of osteophytosis at that specific level of the foramen. Infrequently the foramen may enlarge as a result of an active, progressive lesion. Figures 4-14 and 4-15 are examples of normal oblique views.

Lateral View

The lateral view of the cervical spine is usually the most informative of the standard-routine views of the cervical spine. For this reason, it is best viewed after a thorough, meticulous evaluation of the previous four projections to avoid drawing premature conclusions. Often the lateral view will serve to corroborate the differential established during the review of the previous routine views.

Alignment

The initial assessment of the lateral view of the cervical spine consists of an evaluation of the "overall" alignment of this portion of the spine. Note the existence of an "absence of lordosis" or flattened cervical spine (muscle spasm from trauma), kyphosis (from an anterior segmental compression fracture—Denis's column 1) or a normal-appearing cervical spine with normal lordosis (Figure 4-16 compared to the straightened spine in Figure 4-17.)

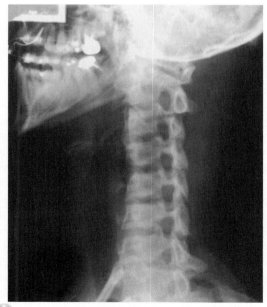

Figure 4-14. ■ Left oblique view of the cervical spine. The oblique view is designed to evaluate the intervertebral foramen. Note the rather consistent size of the foramen throughout the various levels of the cervical spine.

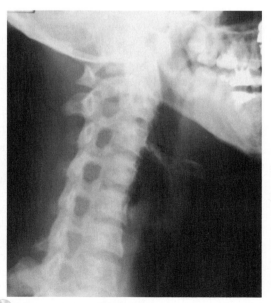

Figure 4-15. ■ Right oblique view of the cervical spine in a normal individual. This view is designed to evaluate the intervertebral foramen.

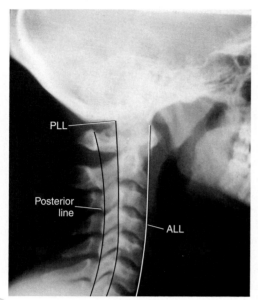

Figure 4-16. ■ **Lateral view of the cervical spine of a normal individual.** Note the alignment of the anterior and posterior vertebral bodies, which should be in a smooth lordotic curve. Bone density of the vertebral bodies, arches, and spinous processes should be consistent. Bone dimensions of the vertebral bodies should be approximately equal between the anterior and posterior bodies. Cartilage spaces should be equal from level to level.

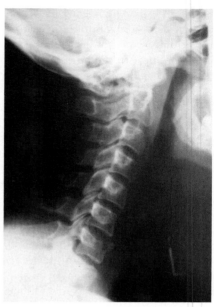

Figure 4-17. ■ **Lateral view of the cervical spine.** Note that the usual lordotic curve is missing, suggesting spasm of the cervical muscles.

The first landmark on the lateral view that requires specific note is the atlantodens interval (ADI). This space measured with a millimeter scale *must not exceed 3 mm*. Any distance greater than 3 mm must be evaluated immediately by a physician for C1 to C2 stability. Instability at this level is clinically manifested by clinical symptoms, such as "when I look down, my head and neck kind of 'clunk'" and/or "my fingers and toes tingle when I look down." These are clearly ominous symptoms that mandate immediate radiologic evaluation and medical treatment. Any patient with a history of significant cervical trauma or a connective tissue/autoimmune disease, such as RA, juvenile rheumatoid arthritis (JRA), systemic lupus erythematosus, or a congenital disease, such as Down syndrome, that puts this C1 to C2 level at risk must have flexion-extension studies done under the controlled guidance of a radiologist. Manual therapy is ruled out as an option until after these studies are performed (Figures 4-18 and 4-19).

The alignment in the cervical spine is evaluated on the lateral projection by drawing lines from superior to inferior along the following structures: anterior longitudinal ligament (ALL), the posterior longitudinal ligament (PLL), and

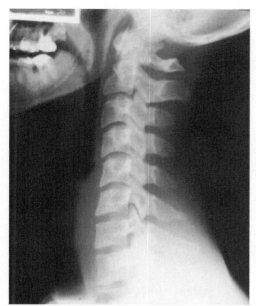

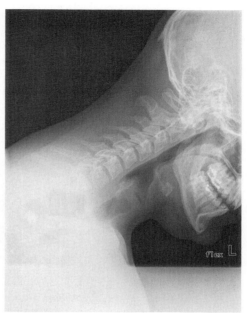

Figure **4-18. ■ Lateral view of the cervical spine allows us to see the ADI, which is the almost vertical line approximately 5 mm posterior to the anterior portion of C1.** This represents the space between the C1 ring and the odontoid process. This space should never exceed 3 mm. It also should not widen with cervical flexion.

Figure **4-19. ■ Lateral view of the cervical spine was taken with the patient's neck in full flexion.** Note that the ADI does not widen with cervical flexion unless there is trauma or a pathologic condition, such as RA that would compromise the connective tissue restraints on C1, allowing it to sublux anteriorly with cervical flexion.

along a line created by the junctions of the lamina and the spinous processes. The ALL and PLL must be parallel, and the posterior line must be consistent—without posterior displacement of any segments. Refer to Figure 4-17 and compare it with Figure 4-18.

If one of the cervical vertebrae is anterior or posterior to these lines, it is an indication of potential instability at that level. In certain types of fracture or soft tissue damage, a portion of one segment will appear to be slightly anterior to the ALL and PLL and yet the laminar-spinous process line will be posterior to the segments above and below. This may indicate a fracture of the pedicle(s), a potential "hangman's fracture," or laminar fracture at that segmental level. Figure 4-20 depicts an x-ray film of a hangman's fracture in the pedicle of C2 with columnar changes: columns one and two are forward, and column three is posterior.

Bone Density and Dimension

Bone is assessed on the lateral projection of the cervical spine by evaluating the density of the vertebral bodies and comparing this with the other cervical vertebrae. Changes in density may indicate disease processes, such as osteoporo-

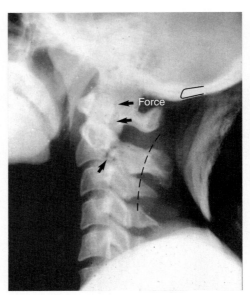

Figure **4-20.** ■ **Lateral view of a patient who had suffered cervical trauma.** Note that the anterior body of C2 overhangs C3. Also the line connecting the posterior cervical bodies is disrupted at C2. A lucency is seen through the pedicles of C2 indicating a fracture. This is known as a "hangman's fracture."

sis, osteolytic or osteoblastic processes, hormonal imbalances, or fractures. Figure 4-21 is a cervical spine film that demonstrates changes in alignment: (1) The ADI is less than 3 mm. (2) There is no displacement anteriorly of the anterior margins of the vertebral bodies along the ALL. There is no posterior displacement of the vertebral bodies when compared with the segments above and below along the PLL. (3) There is evidence that Denis's column three is shifted posteriorly along a lucent line that is through the pedicles of C2. This is a hangman's fracture.

Figure 4-22 is a film of a 27-year-old male with ankylosing spondylitis. This disease, which is thought to be an autoimmune disease with a slight familial component, first becomes symptomatic in the lumbosacral joint(s). There is evidence of syndesmophytes bridging the anterior vertebral bodies and ossifications of the annulus fibrosis, giving this the name "bamboo spine." The uncinate joints are involved in column two. It is also occasionally referred to as Marie-Strümpell disease.[9]

Dimensions can be measured anterior to posterior (horizontally) along the superior and inferior margins of the vertebral bodies from C3 to C7 and superior to inferior along the ALL and PLL in millimeters. Changes in dimensions may indicate a column one or two collapse of a vertebrae as a result of trauma or osteoporosis, (pathologic fracture), congenital malformation, osteophytosis, etc. (Figure 4-23).

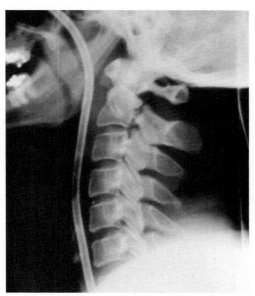

Figure 4-21. ■ **The ADI interval is less than 3 mm, which is normal.** The alignment of the anterior and posterior cervical vertebral bodies is normal. However, the posterior column (the spinous process) is seen to be posterior. Additionally there is a fracture through the pedicles. This is also a "hangman's fracture," but without displacement of the body.

Cartilage

Assessment of cartilage in the cervical spine, as elsewhere in the spine, entails assessments of the intervertebral disks. Pathologic conditions in the disks are divided into diseases of the annulus fibrosis, such as enthesis (inflammation of the Sharpey's fibers) osteoarthritis, and diseases of the nucleus pulposus: herniated nucleus pulposus (HNP), diskitis—normally an infection of the disk relegated to younger patients, etc. Infrequently, when an HNP occurs, over time, nitrogen will move from the cartilaginous endplates of the vertebral bodies into the potential space created by the evacuation of the nucleus pulposus and will be visible as an area of decreased density within the confines of the intervertebral space and is known as a "vacuum phenomenon." This is seen more frequently in the lumbar spine, but it can occur in the cervical spine.[10]

Soft Tissue

Soft tissue is evaluated in several areas of the cervical spine. Anterior to the vertebral bodies and the ALL is the prevertebral tissue. An area of decreased density in this region may be indicative of hemorrhage from an occult fracture of the vertebrae that is immediately posterior to the lucency. An increased distance between the spinous processes may indicate a tear of the interspinal ligament and supraspinal ligament, indicating potentially severe segmental instability. Overall "flattening" of the normal cervical lordosis is an indication of

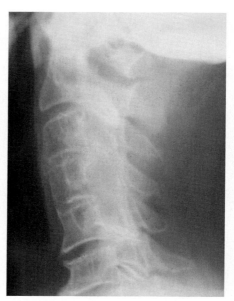

Figure 4-22. ■ **Lateral cervical view of a 27-year-old male with ankylosing spondylitis.** Note the syndesmophytes bridging the anterior vertebral bodies and the ossification of the annulus fibrosis. The uncinate joints are also fused at the C3 to C5 level by the disease.

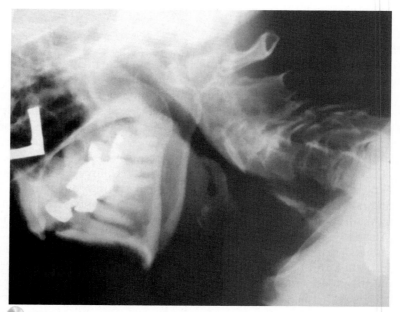

Figure 4-23. ■ **Lateral cervical view of a 72-year-old female with RA.** Note the decreased mineralization of the cervical spine and the anterior subluxation of C4 on C5.

cervical spasm. This is generally a nonspecific finding indicating cervical spasm, which accompanies most cervical insults from muscle spasm to fracture and instability. Figure 4-24 depicts a loss of lordosis, which is often caused by cervical spasm. An additional finding is a decreased disk space at the C3-4 level and a possible incomplete segmentation at this level in columns one and two.

Instabilities: Evaluation of soft tissue mandates a consideration of the integrity of the connective tissue. Following trauma or a significant disease that may compromise the connective tissue, it is possible to have a dislocation of the spine without fracturing the bones of the spine, which increases the risk of catastrophic results (Figure 4-25). Figure 4-26 demonstrates what is most likely an old compression fracture of C6 in column 1; it also demonstrates an alarming increase in the excursion of the inferior articular facets of C5 on the superior articular facets on C6 with the real potential of a dislocation and the potential neurologic damage associated with this event. Although this is categorized under soft tissue, it could also be considered an alignment finding. Rockwood, Green, and Bucholz distinguish between the categories of flexion, extension, and rotational instability in the spine.[11] There is a predictable pattern of trauma and combinations of movements that result in specific instabilities. Flexion instability can result from ligamentous incompetency or a combination of bony instability and ligamentous incompetentcy.[11]

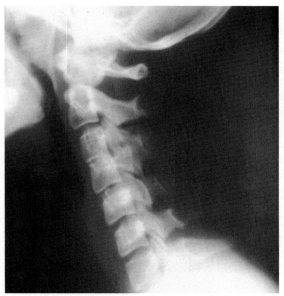

Figure 4-24. ■ Depicts a loss of lordosis, which is often caused by cervical spasm. An additional finding is a decreased disk space at C3-4 and a possible incomplete segmentation at this level in columns two and three of C3 to C4.

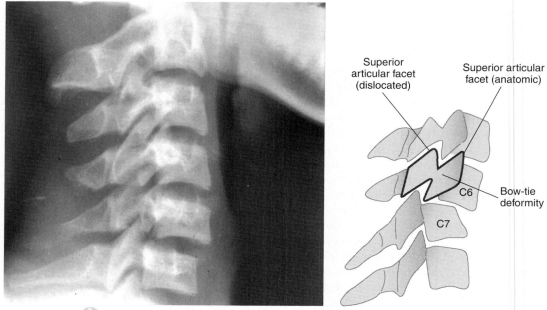

Figure 4-25. ■ **Depicts a dislocation of C5 with anterior displacement of the vertebral body.** *(From Marx JA:* Rosen's Emergency Medicine, *ed 6, St. Louis, Mosby 2006)*

Variations on "Normal"

The skeletal system has many variations on the normal, and they are much too numerous to address in this introductory volume, but a few will be noted.

The absence of space between two vertebral bodies may represent a herniation of the nucleus pulposus, or another explanation may be a failure of embryonic segmentation at one or multiple levels. Figure 4-27 demonstrates a failure of segmentation at the C4 to C5 vertebral body. Segmentation failures run the gamut from a failure to completely segment, partial segmentation, and incomplete closure (spina bifida occulta) to completely open and exposed lower vertebral neural elements in the more severely involved individuals with spina bifida. Others may take the form of "block vertebrae," "hemivertebrae," or transitional vertebrae (there is one classification for six variations on this anomaly alone).[12] These aberrations may be most visible on AP views or lateral views. A lack of complete segmentation should be considered in the differential diagnosis in the absence of other obvious explanations for chronic cervical pain, especially in atraumatic cases that have not been x-rayed and on examination have specific segments that are completely immobile. These diagnoses may respond to soft tissue rehabilitation, but aggressive manual therapy is not recommended on these nonmobile segment levels. These nonsegmented spinal units may be found throughout the spine from the cervical level to the lumbosacral level.

Test your understanding by taking a quiz on this chapter with the accompanying DVD.

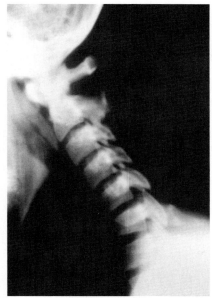

Figure 4-26. ■ **Note that the anterior body of C6 is not as high as the posterior body.** This is a compression fracture. Also the articular facet "shingling" of C5 on C6 is much more open than the other levels, with the real potential of a dislocation with the potential neurologic damage associated with that event.

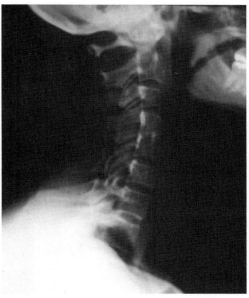

Figure 4-27. ■ **Lateral view of the cervical spine.** Note the absence of space between the vertebral bodies of C4 and C5. This represents a failure of segmentation of C4 and C5.

CASE STUDIES

CASE STUDY A

"Sometimes the most important things you see are what you cannot see!": Figures 4-28 to 4-31 are films of a 21-year-old college student with a history of unilateral pain and progressive weakness in his ipsilateral triceps who was referred to physical therapy with "neck pain." The patient was treated for 10 days and referred back to the orthopedic surgeon with "no improvement and increasing weakness." The patient was referred back to the physical therapy clinic for more therapy after standard-plain films were taken of the patient's neck and read as normal by a radiologist. The patient was seen for another 2 weeks in therapy and then went home from college for Christmas break. While at home, the patient sought the opinion of his hometown physician and was referred to a neurosurgical physician for definitive care. The only finding is of a "slight indistinctness" on the right as we view the film at the C7 root level (Figure 4-28). This is not normally a significant finding unless it corroborates suspicions from the history and physical examination. Figure 4-29 depicts an oblique view of the noninvolved side. The x-ray film depicted normal findings with equal intervertebral foramina. An oblique view of the symptomatic side demonstrates clearly the "jacked open" intervertebral foramen at the C7 root level (Figure 4-30). It is especially significant when correlated with the signs and symptoms and compared with the opposite or noninvolved side. This was the result of a schwannoma at the nerve root of C7. It was debulked by a neurosurgeon, and the patient's pain was resolved. His reflex at that level did not return, and his triceps on the ipsilateral side tested at the "trace" (1/5) level. Figure 4-31 is a lateral view of the patient's cervical spine. There is clearly an increased dimension of the C7 foramen just anterior to the facets, particularly when compared with the levels above and below.

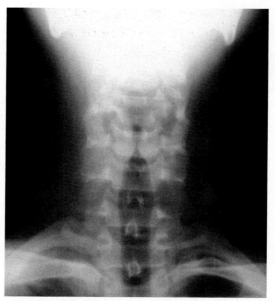

Figure **4-28.** ■ **Film of a 21-year-old college student with a history of unilateral pain and progressive weakness in the ipsilateral triceps muscle without a history of trauma.** On the AP view, alignment, bone, and soft tissue appear normal. Cartilage is not well visualized on the AP view.

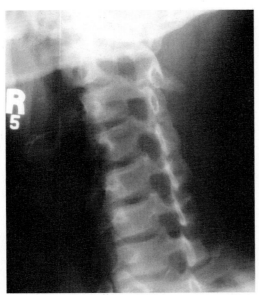

Figure 4-29. ■ **Right oblique cervical view of the same individual shown in Figures 4-28 to 4-31.** Alignment, bone, cartilage, and soft tissue appear normal.

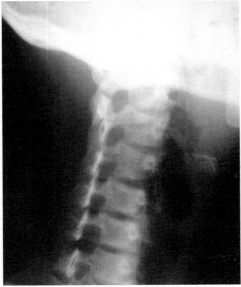

Figure 4-30. ■ **Left oblique view.** All findings appear normal, except that the foramen for cervical root 7 appears to be larger than the others. The C7 root findings correlated with the patient's complaint of pain and weakness in the triceps muscle. At surgery, the patient was found to have a schwannoma that was growing in the foramen. The schwannoma was forcing the joint open and strangling the C7 nerve root.

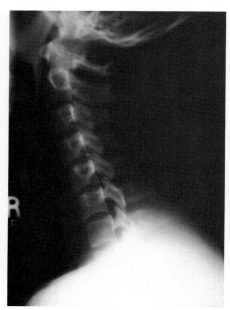

Figure 4-31. ■ **Lateral view of the cervical spine of the patient shown in Figures 4-28 to 4-31.** The C6-C7 foramen is visibly larger than those above, even in this view.

CASE STUDY B

Using imaging modalities to guide evidence-based decision processes: Figures 4-32 to 4-34 are films of a 22-year-old male who, while on a visit to his rural home during a break from college, dove into a pond and struck his head on an underwater object. He experienced an immediate onset of neck spasm and pain. He went to his hometown physician who x-rayed his neck and, although concerned, recommended that the student follow up with the "experts" at the university. The patient was a football player who wanted to return to his sport as soon as possible. His examination was normal for strength and neurologic signs and symptoms in his upper extremities. His routine-plain films were:

Open mouth: normal
AP: normal
Obliques: normal
Lateral (Figure 4-32):

Alignment: This film demonstrates a loss of cervical lordosis. There is an actual kyphotic section at the C5 level. There are no vertebrae displaced anteriorly or posteriorly when the ALL and PLL are carefully checked.

Bone dimensions: There is a decrease in the AP dimension at the superior level of C5 and an accompanying decrease in the superior and/or inferior dimension anteriorly at C5.

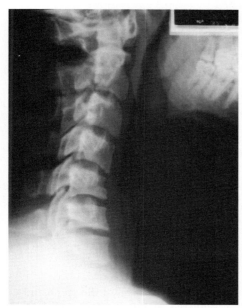

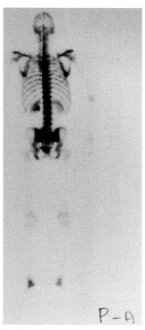

Figure 4-32. ■ **Lateral view of a 22-year-old male who dove into a pond and struck his head.** He had an immediate onset of neck spasm and pain. Three weeks later, he went back to college where he was a football player. He wants to play football next week. His strength and neurologic signs are normal. Note the decreased height of the anterior vertebral body of C5.

Figure 4-33. ■ **This image is a bone scan of the 22-year-old patient in Figure 4-32.** The entire spine indicates rapid bone activity, as do the shoulders and heels. There is too much activity to make judgments about the cervical spine.

Cartilage: Cartilage is well maintained at all levels.

Soft tissue: No soft tissue changes can be appreciated.

The diagnosis was a compression fracture of the anterior-superior vertebral body of C5. No evidence of instability was found during motion studies. At this point, we have a college athlete who competes in a collision sport with a history of an acute neck injury. He has an x-ray film finding of a small, stable fracture of the C5 vertebral body and wants to return to play sports as soon as possible. The question then is, "is this a new or old injury." The decision was made to perform a bone scan on this patient to assess the metabolic activity at this level, and if the bone was metabolically more active than the surrounding cervical vertebrae, the patient would have to sit out the season. The patient agreed to this.

The bone scan (Figure 4-33):

This view is not particularly informative because it is too active and not specific enough to answer the question. The radiologist who knew the question to be answered has provided a "dialed down" (remember that in bone scanning sometimes "less is more") version that addressed the specific head and neck region.

The views of the lower back, pelvis, AP of head and neck, and lateral of the head and neck clearly show that the C5 vertebra is metabolically more active than the

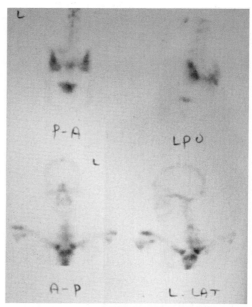

🔵 *Figure* 4-34. ■ **This image is a lower power scan of the spine and shoulder areas of the individual depicted in Figures 4-32 and 4-33.** Note that there is evidence of active bone metabolism at the C5 level. This individual still has active healing in the cervical spine area and should not yet return to sports.

surrounding vertebrae, and the decision was made to hold this athlete out that year (Figure 4-34). Remember that the radiopharmaceutical is cleared from the blood by the kidneys and the bladder will always be active.

CASE STUDY C

Cervical Spine: A 72-year-old female with a long history of RA and multiple comorbidities was referred to physical therapy for evaluation and treatment of chronic neck pain. The patient was not a surgical candidate and had a long history of prescription prednisone use. On examination she had severely limited range of motion (ROM) of the cervical spine and had radicular symptoms accompanying ROM measurements and motor testing. She was neurologically intact, and motor strength was symmetrical in both upper extremities (BUE). She rated her pain as 9/10. She had multiple involvements in multiple other joints, as would be expected with this duration of the diagnosis of RA.

Her lateral cervical spine film is shown in Figure 4-27.

The patient's age and long history of prednisone use have left her vertebrae severely osteoporotic. Her ADI is greater than 3 mm. This view does not visualize C7, and no routine-plain film study of the cervical spine is complete without visualizing the complete cervical spine including C7 (see Figure 4-23).

Alignment: With a long history of an autoimmune disease such as RA you would expect severe damage to the connective tissue resulting in multiple levels of instability, and there are multiple examples of malalignment in this patient's cervical vertebrae: The C2 vertebra is rotated in an axial plane to the point where you can visualize portions of both sides of the pedicles and the laminae. The C3 vertebra is anteriorly displaced on C4 and is rotated clockwise as we view this film. C4 is displaced anteriorly on C5.

Bone density: The entire spine is severely osteoporotic.

Dimensions: The dimensions are acceptable.

Cartilage: C3 has stretched the anterior annulus. Although not visible on routine films, the annulus does not normally permit the visible distortion(s) presented on this view. C5 has collapsed onto C6 and clearly has herniated its nuclear contents.

Soft tissue: There is evidence of calcification anterior to the lower cervical spine. This *may* represent carotid calcification.

The last, rather ominous, information that is not evident on this lateral film, because most markings were removed for the patient's privacy, is that this was an extension film in a series of motion studies to assess the stability of her cervical spine.

REFERENCES

1. Streitwieser D et al: Accuracy of standard radiographic views in detecting cervical spine fractures, *Ann Emerg Med* 12:538-542, 1983.
2. Rockwood CA, Green DP, Bucholz RW: *Fractures in adults,* ed 3, Philadelphia, 1991, Lippincott Williams & Wilkins.
3. Bosh A, Stauffer ES, Nickel VL: Incomplete traumatic quadriplegia: a ten year review, *JAMA* 216:473-478, 1971.
4. Bradford DS, Thompson RC: Fractures and dislocations of the spine, *Minn Med* 59:711-720, 1976.
5. Bohlman HH: Acute fractures and dislocations of the cervical spine, *JBJS* 61A:1119-1142, 1979.
6. Rockwood CA, Green DP: *Fractures in adults,* Philadelphia, 1991, Lippincott Williams & Wilkins.
7. Denis F: The three-column spine and its significance in the classification of acute thoracolumbar spinal injuries, *Spine* 8:817-831, 1983.
8. Allen BL: Recognition of injuries to the lower cervical spine. In Cervical Spine Research Committee, editor: *The cervical spine,* Philadelphia, 1989, JB Lippincott.
9. Greenspan A: *Orthopedic radiology,* ed 2, New York, Raven Press.
10. Bohrer SP, Chen YM: Cervical spine annulus vacuum, *Skeletal Radiol* 17(5):324-329.
11. Rockwood CA, Green DP: *Fractures in adults,* Philadelphia, 1991, Lippincott Williams & Wilkins.
12. Brenner AK: Use of lumbosacral region manipulation and therapeutic exercises for a patient with a lumbosacral transitional vertebra and low back pain, *JOSPT* 35(6):368-376.
13. Rockwood CA, Green DP: *Fractures in adults,* ed 3, vol 2, Philadelphia, 1991, Lippincott Williams & Wilkins.

5 The Lumbar Spine

INTRODUCTION

Remarks

The five vertebrae that comprise the lumbar spine are similar to the rest of the vertebrae in the spine in the overall shape, components, and relative alignment of the individual vertebrae. The individual vertebrae are larger than the cephalad thoracic and cervical vertebrae, and the articular surfaces of the facets are oriented in a sagittal direction. When compared with the individual vertebral segments above (cephalad), the lumbar spinous processes are shorter, thicker, and often not visible on the "lateral" projection. The lumbar spine is at risk for the same diseases, tumors, instabilities, and fractures as the rest of the skeletal system.

When initially viewing the lumbar spine films, count down the vertebrae and identify that there are five lumbar vertebrae, as opposed to four as found in "sacralization" of L5 or six as found in "lumbarization" of the first sacral segment (Figure 5-1). Note any variations and apply the ABCS.

OBJECTIVES

1. Recall the five standard lumbar spine views and their purposes.
2. Identify normal and pathologic alignment of the five standard views.
3. Identify normal and pathologic densities and dimensions of lumbar spine bones.
4. Identify normal and pathologic cartilage.
5. Identify normal and pathologic presentation of soft tissue.
6. Given a history and x-ray film, identify film abnormalities.
7. Given x-ray film abnormalities, use that information to adjust a physical therapy treatment program.

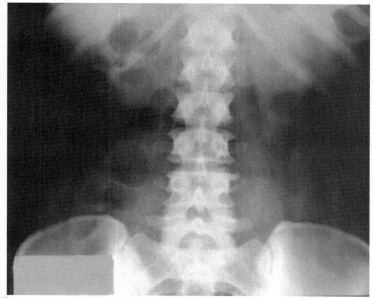

Figure 5-1. ■ Lumbarization of S1. Count down the lumbar verte-brae from L1 (the one below the last rib) and note that there are appar-ently six lumbar vertebrae. Alignment is acceptable.

STANDARD VIEWS

There are five separate views required to perform the basic evaluation of the lumbar spine with plain film x-rays:
1. Anteroposterior (AP) (Figure 5-2)
2. Left oblique (Figure 5-3)
3. Right oblique (Figure 5-3)
4. Lateral (Figure 5-4)
5. "Coned-down view" of lumbosacral joint (Figure 5-5)

It may be helpful to view the coned-down view of L5 to S1 as the view unique to the lumbar spine. To properly view this segment, the x-rays must penetrate both sides of the iliac bones, and as a result, it subjects the patient to the highest dosage of rads of any of the standard-plain film views and should be used judiciously.

EVALUATION OF THE LUMBAR SPINE USING ABCS

Anteroposterior

Identification of the anatomical landmarks in the AP view of the lumbar spine is more easily done if this view is thought of as a Native American "totem pole." The figures on the totem represent the heads of large predatory birds, raptors that are looking straight at you. Think eagles, hawks, or owls. The

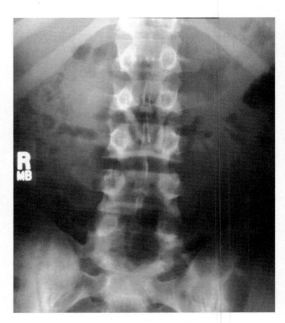

Figure 5-2. ■ **Alignment is acceptable.** Pedicles can be assessed to evaluate rotation. *Bone:* dimensions are acceptable. *Density:* the laminae of L5 do not fuse into one spinous process. This is known as "spina bifida occulta." This is the mildest form of spina bifida, a failure of complete segmentation embryologically.

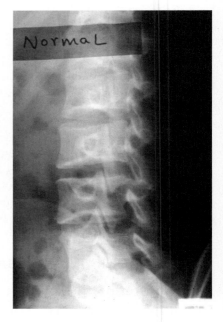

Figure 5-3. ■ **Example of a normal oblique view of the lumbar spine.** Obliques in the lumbar spine are specifically designed to evaluate the status of the pars interarticularis. It is the "neck" of the "Scottie dog." If the dog's neck has a lucency through it, that is diagnostic of spondylolysis. Spondylolysis can be unilateral or bilateral and found at one or several levels. It is most common at L5 and less so at L4.

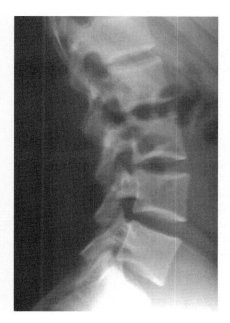

Figure 5-4. ■ **Standard lateral view of the lumbar spine.** Alignment, bone (density and dimensions) are excellent, cartilage (disk spaces) is well maintained, and soft tissue is normally poorly visualized in the lumbar spine projections.

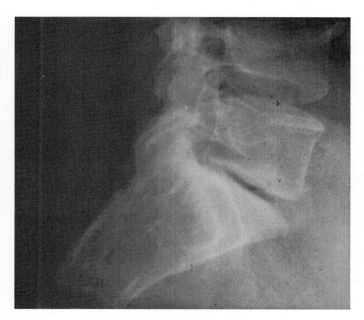

Figure 5-5. ■ This coned-down view of the L5-S1 interspace and vertebral bodies shows excellent alignment; however, the L5-S1 interspace is markedly decreased when compared with the L4-L5 level above. The L5-S1 interspace has a lucency (darkened region between the vertebral bodies) that is known as a "vacuum phenomenon."

vertebral body represents the bird's head, the pedicles the bird's eyes, transverse processes are feathers from the bird's head, and the lamina and the spinous processes form the bird's beak. Refer to Figure 5-2 and identify all the parts at all five levels. *Note:* Carefully identify all of the pedicles of the lumbar and thoracic spine (usually T12 is visible). Certain metastatic processes have a predilection for the vertebral pedicles, darkening one "eye" and resulting in what Dr. Resnick referred to as the "winking owl.[1]"

Alignment

The assessment of alignment in the AP view of the lumbar spine relies upon the following bony landmarks: the spinous processes should align vertically. If they do not align vertically, it is an indication of rotation at one or more segments. Do the lateral surfaces of the vertebral bodies line up vertically, or is/are there lateral displacement(s) to the left or right at one or more levels? Mentally draw horizontal lines left to right across the superior and inferior vertebral end plates and look for parallel lines. An angle formed by one of these lines may indicate a unilateral compression fracture or osteoporotic collapse of a portion of the vertebral body. If the lack of parallelism is a result of scoliosis rather than a disease process or fracture, there is usually rotation accompanying the change as indicated by a displacement of the spinous process and shift in the pedicles, as is seen in Figure 5-6.

Bone Density and Dimension

Figure 5-7 demonstrates the "double lamina" sign of a severe spondylolisthesis caused by the inferior, or caudal, displacement of L5 on S1 when viewed in an AP plane.

Left and Right Oblique Views (Figure 5-8)

The obliques are taken with the patient supine and the shoulders and lower spine and pelvis rotated toward the side to be imaged (Figure 5-9), left obliques with the left side elevated and right obliques with the right side rotated from the supine position. The obliques are used to image a spondylolysis (Figures 5-10 to 5-13). To visualize this, envision a Scottie dog where:

Pedicles = Scottie dog's eye.

Articular facets = superior facet is the Scottie dog's ear, inferior is the Scottie dog's front legs, superior facet on opposite side is the Scottie dog's tail, and the inferior articular facet on the opposite side is the Scottie dog's back legs.

Transverse processes = Scottie dog's muzzle.

Pars interarticularis = represented by Scottie dog's neck. If there is a lucency through the Scottie dog's neck (the Scottie dog is "wearing a collar"), it represents a fracture of the pars interarticularis.

Lateral View (see Figure 5-4)

Alignment

Spondylolisthesis: Is the anterior vertebral body vertically aligned with the vertebral body below (see Figure 5-10)? These are graded by the percent of displacement or "overhang": grade 1 is 25% displacement, grade 2 is 50% displacement, grade 3 is 75% displacement, and grade 4 is greater than 75% displacement (Figures 5-14 to 5-18).

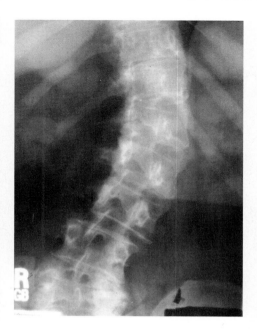

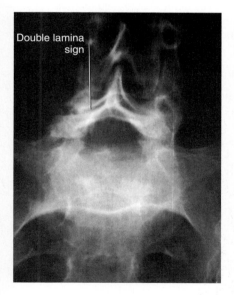

Double lamina sign

Figure **5-6. ■ AP of the lumbar spine.** Alignment is unacceptable. L3 is shifted to the L on L4. The step off is obvious on the L and R sides of the spine. The curve is convex to the R, and the concavity is to the L. Rotation begins at L3 on L4 inferiorly and ends at T11 proximally when the spinous processes and pedicles are used to measure rotation on this view. *Bone:* the vertebral bodies demonstrate decreased density indicating osteoporosis. Cartilage would be better assessed on the lateral view. Soft tissue is not well visualized.

Figure **5-7. ■ AP of the lumbosacral junction.** There is bilateral spondylolysis *(arrow 1)*, and the laminae of L5 appear to be in close proximity to those of S1, the "double lamina sign" *(arrow 2)*. The laminae appear to be in such close proximity because L5 has slid anteriorly and inferiorly on S1. This movement forward on one spinal segment anteriorly on the segment below it is called *spondylolisthesis*. This figure is an AP of a grade L4-L5 on S1 spondylolisthesis.

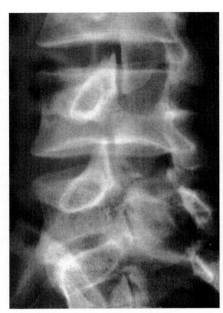

Figure 5-8. ■ **Oblique tomogram (magnified plain x-ray) that demonstrates a spondylolysis at L5-S1.** The additional finding on this film is that L4-L5 also has a fracture through the pars interarticularis, reinforcing the necessity to evaluate the films in a systematic, disciplined manner to prevent overlooking additional pathologic conditions by becoming too fixed on the obvious pathologic conditions.

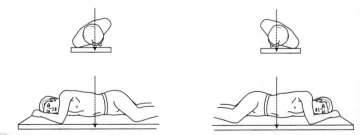

Figure 5-9. ■ **Patient positioning for an oblique lumbar x-ray.** *(From Long BW, Frank ED, Ehrlich RA:* Radiography essentials for limited practice, *ed 2, 2006, Saunders.)*

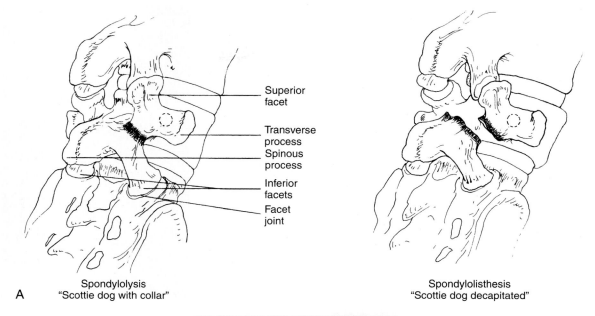

Superior
facet

Transverse
process

Spinous
process

Inferior
facets

Facet
joint

A

Spondylolysis
"Scottie dog with collar"

Spondylolisthesis
"Scottie dog decapitated"

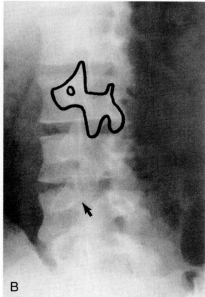

B

Figure 5-10. ■ **A,** Diagrammatic representation (posterior oblique view) of spondylolysis and spondylolisthesis. **B,** Posterior oblique film showing "Scottie dog" at L2. L4 shows Scottie dog with a "collar" *(arrow),* indicating spondylolysis. *(From Magee DJ:* Orthopedic physical assessment enhanced edition, *ed 4, Philadelphia, 2006, Saunders.)*

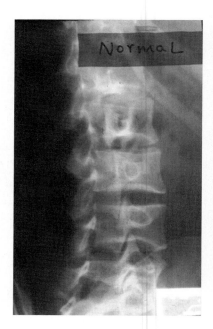

Figure 5-11. ■ Obliques of the lumbar spine. No significant bony pathologic conditions noted. Identify the nose, eye, ear, front, and back leg of the "Scottie dog" and compare it with the anatomical drawings shown in Figure 5-10.

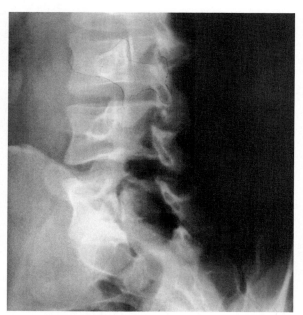

Figure 5-12. ■ **Oblique of the lumbar spine.** Note the dark "collar" that is indicative of an L5-S1 spondylolysis.

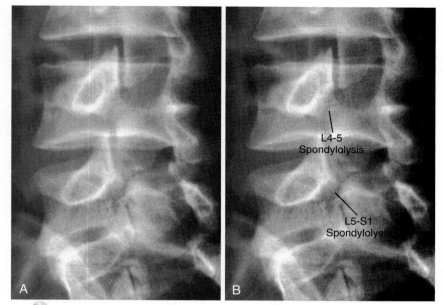

🔘 *Figure* 5-13. ▪ **What do you see on the film (A)?** Compare it with the tomogram (**B**). Note that there are two levels of spondylolysis, at L4-L5 and at L5-S1.

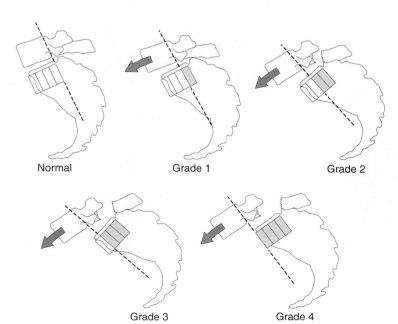

🔘 *Figure* 5-14. ▪ **This figure depicts the grading system for determining the severity of spondylolisthesis.** Each grade represents a 25% slippage, with a grade 1 up to 25%, grade 2 from 25% to 50%, grade 3 50% to 75%, and grade 4 greater than 75% slippage. (*From Magee DJ:* Orthopedic physical assessment enhanced edition, *ed 4, Philadelphia, 2006, Saunders.*)

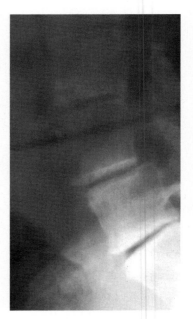

Figure **5-15.** ■ Note the grade 1 L4 on L5 spondylolisthesis.

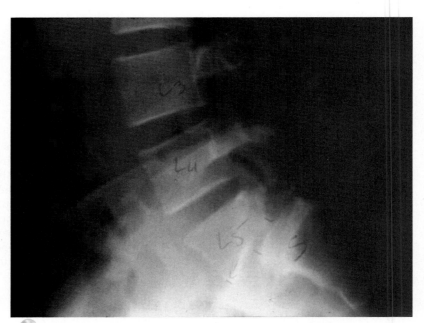

Figure **5-16.** ■ This figure depicts a 50% forward slippage of L5 on S1, which is a grade 2 or 3 spondylolisthesis.

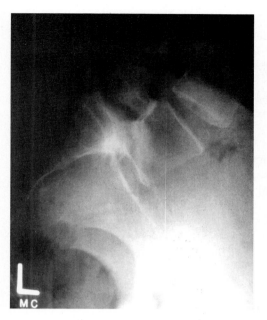

Figure 5-17. ■ **The overlay of the iliac bones makes it more difficult to initially see the extreme slippage in this view.** The sacrum is in the upper left quadrant of this film with the posterior portion of the L5 vertebral body slipped forward more than 75%, making this a grade 3 to 4 spondylolisthesis. Note the erosion of the posterior inferior portion of L5 and the eburnation of the interface of L5 and S1. Note that to achieve this displacement, the entire annulus and the major stabilizing ligaments of the spine must be compromised.

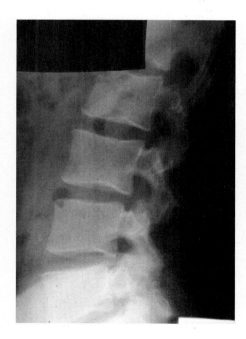

Figure 5-18. ■ **Although it is much less common, it is possible for the superior portion of the spinal column to move posterior on the more inferior body.** Note in this Figure that L4 has moved posterior to the L5 body, creating a grade 1 retrolisthesis at L5-S1.

Coned-Down View

The coned-down view is a lateral view of the L5-S1 joint with the x-ray energy so high that the iliac crests become invisible (see Figure 5-5). The lumbar and sacral bodies can then be visualized.

Alignment

Is the inferior portion of the L5 body aligned with the superior body of S1? Note in Figure 5-16 that L5 is approximately one third forward with respect to the S1 body.

Bone Density and Dimension

Density: The quality of the L5 bone is checked.

Dimensions: Dimensions in the superior-inferior and anteroposterior planes should be approximately equal.

Cartilage

The intervertebral space, or disk space, is checked for a vacuum phenomenon.

Soft Tissue

Soft tissue is not visible as a result of the high dosage of radiation, which renders the soft tissue invisible.

Variations on "Normal"

The skeletal system has many variations on the normal, and they are much too numerous to address in this introductory volume, but a few will be noted.

The absence of space between two vertebral bodies may represent a herniation of the nucleus pulposus, or another explanation may be a failure of embryonic segmentation at one or more levels, as shown in Figure 5-19. They run the gamut from a failure to completely segment, partial segmentation, and

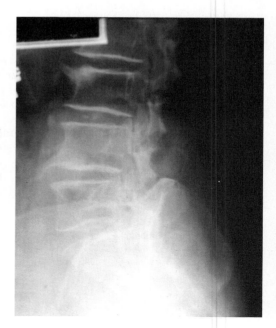

Figure 5-19. ■ A lateral view of the lumbosacral spine with sponlylosis deformans. Note the well preserved disk spaces and significant spurring of the anterior body. This is a calcification of Sharpey's fibers.

incomplete closure (spina bifida occulta) to completely open and exposed lower vertebral neural elements in the more severely involved babies with spina bifida. Others may take the form of "block vertebrae," "hemivertebrae," or transitional vertebrae (there is one classification for six variations on this anomaly alone).[2] These aberrations may be most visible on AP views or lateral views. In the absence of other obvious explanations for chronic spine pain, especially in atraumatic cases that have not been x-rayed and on examination have specific segments that are completely immobile, lack of complete segmentation should be considered in the differential. These diagnoses may respond to soft tissue rehabilitation, but aggressive manual therapy is not recommended on these nonmobile segment levels. These nonsegmented spinal units are found throughout the spine from the cervical level to the lumbosacral level.

Test your understanding by taking a quiz on this chapter.

CASE STUDIES

CASE STUDY A

History: The patient is a 23-year-old female married to a graduate physical therapy student. She is an active runner of marathons who has chronic nonradicular low back pain. She is planning on starting a family, but is not presently pregnant. She has requested evaluation of her low back pain before her pregnancy.

Physical Findings: Normal deep tendon reflexes (DTRs), strength, and lower extremity range of motion (ROM). Decreased side bending and flexion noted.

Imaging:

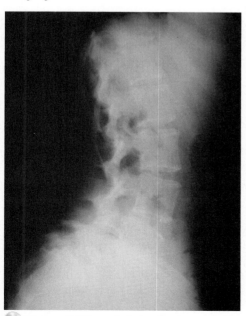

Image: Figure 5-20
Your impressions:
1. Alignment
2. Bone density and dimension
3. Cartilage
4. Soft tissue

Figure 5-20. ■ A lateral view of the lumbosacral spine.

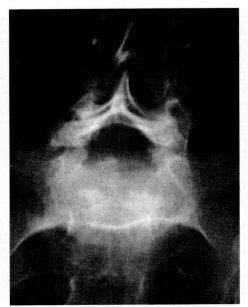

Figure **5-21.** ■ **Coned-down AP view of L5-S1.**

Image: Figure 5-21
Your impressions:
1. Alignment
2. Bone density and dimension
3. Cartilage
4. Soft tissue

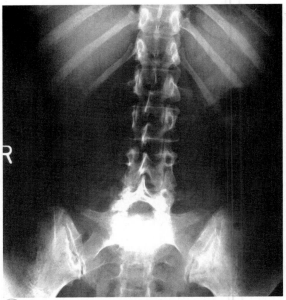

Figure **5-22.** ■ **AP view of the lumbar spine demonstrating the double lamina sign of severe spondylolisthesis.**

Image: Figure 5-22
Your impressions:
1. Alignment
2. Bone density and dimension
3. Cartilage
4. Soft tissue

Our Impressions: The patient has grade 3 spondylolisthesis of L5 on S1. The AP demonstrates a "double lamina" sign, and there is a spondylolysis visible on the AP and the "zoomed in" AP. The lateral view demonstrates clearly that at times the coned-down view is required to adequately visualize the L5-S1 segment.

Therapy Questions:
A. What treatment would you suggest for the patient?
B. If the patient asked whether pregnancy would worsen her back problem, how would you respond?
C. What would be your counsel concerning her continuance of running marathons?

CASE STUDY B

History: An 18-year-old female involved in a one-vehicle roll-over accident arrives at the emergency room with severe upper lumbar, lower thoracic back pain. She is neurologically intact.

Physical Findings: A lateral view of the thoracolumbar spine demonstrates an intact bony structure with no fractures (Figure 5-23). However, the marked increase in the dimension of the intervertebral foramen at L1-L2 compared with the levels above and below indicates gross instability of the posterior, column three, ligamentous structures.

Figure 5-24 is an intraoperative film with the patient in extension and the instability reduced. Figure 5-25 is an intraoperative film with the internal fixation in place to stabilize the segment while ligamentous healing proceeds.

The patient was sent to physical therapy postoperatively for pain control and strengthening of the paraspinal musculature "appropriate for her condition." She was neurologically intact and had good pain control. She attended two sessions while hospitalized, but after discharge, she never returned to therapy or medical follow-up.

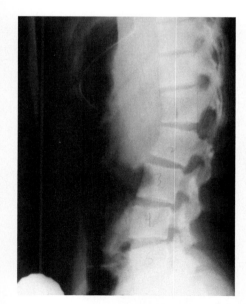

Figure 5-23. ■ **The initial lateral view of the thoracolumbar spine.**

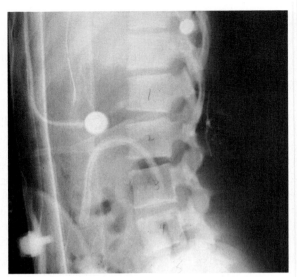

Figure 5-24. ■ The operative lateral view of the thoracolumbar spine.

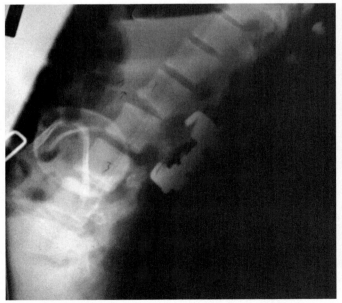

Figure 5-25. ■ An intraoperative lateral view of the fixated thoracolumbar spine.

CASE STUDY C

The patient is an 80 year old female with low back pain of long standing. The patient has multiple medical problems. Back pain radiates down the left hip and across the thigh. Two views; lateral and coned down view. Please state <u>all</u> your findings including soft tissue.

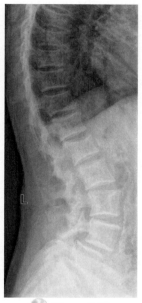

Figure 5-26

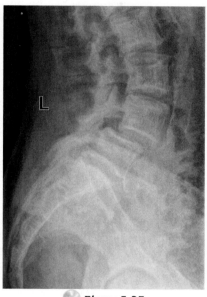

Figure 5-27

Image: Figure 5-26
Your impressions:
1. Alignment
2. Bone density and dimension
3. Cartilage
4. Soft tissue

Image: Figure 5-27
Your impressions:
1. Alignment
2. Bone density and dimension
3. Cartilage
4. Soft tissue

Our impressions:
1. *Alignment*: The L4 body is displaced anterior to the vertebral body of L5 on this lateral view. The patient has a grade I L4 on L5 spondylolisthesis
2. *Bone density and dimension*: Bone density is consistently decreased, indicating advanced osteoporosis
3. *Cartilage*: Lumbar disc space is reasonably well maintained.
4. *Soft tissue*: This patient has marked abdominal aortic calcifications that define the margins of this vessel.

Our impressions: The films reveal unilateral spondylolysis and contralateral sclerosis indicating a high probability of impending fracture through the pars.

The aortic calcifications are a consideration when designing a manual therapy intervention or evaluating the type of exercise program to apply with this patient.
A. How would you treat this patient?
B. What would you suggest for treatment of the back pain?
C. What would you suggest for general conditioning?

Therapy questions: The appropriate therapy intervention, well designed and carefully monitored has the potential to improve this patients mobility and pain. The key is the design and consideration of her comorbidities.

REFERENCES

1. Resnick D, Niwayama G: *Diagnosis of bone and joint disorders,* ed 2, Philadelphia, 1998, Saunders.
2. Brenner AK: Use of lumbosacral region manipulation and therapeutic exercises for a patient with a lumbosacral transitional vertebra and low back pain, *JOSPT* 35(6):368-376.

6 The Hip

INTRODUCTION ▰▰▰▰▰▰▰

Remarks

The hip is unique compared with other major joints in the human skeleton because it is an inherently stable joint when compared, for example, with the inherently unstable shoulder. The femur articulates proximally with the acetabulum, and the shaft of the femur is offset at an angle of 130 degrees (plus or minus 7 degrees) to the acetabulum.[1] The shaft is strong cortical bone that, in a healthy adult, may require up to 1000 lb of shear force to break. From the proximal shaft of the femur, the bone transitions to cancellous bone and travels proximally and medially across the femoral neck, terminating in the rounded femoral head. This structural arrangement places enormous forces across the cervical, or neck, region of the proximal femur. When viewed in an anteroposterior (AP) plane, the proximal femoral neck and head form an angle with the diaphysis of the femur of 125 to 130 degrees.

The pelvis is formed by two iliac wings, which attach posterior medially to the sacrum, the two pubic bones, and the two ischial bones. These three bones join laterally to form the hip socket, or acetabulum. The fusion of the three

99

bones of the hip on each side of the pelvis used to be known as the innominate bone.

As with all joints, imaging of the hip for physical therapists is best employed to understand the pathologic condition or potential pathologic condition and assist in treatment planning by demonstrating the extent of the injury or disease and contraindications to specific exercises and modalities and the levels of each that may be safely administered during the consecutive phases of healing and rehabilitation.

OBJECTIVES

1. Recall the two standard views of the hip joint and their purposes.
2. Identify the normal and abnormal alignment in the standard views of the hip and pelvis.
3. Identify normal and abnormal densities and dimensions of the hip.
4. Identify normal and abnormal cartilage.
5. Identify the normal and abnormal presentation of soft tissue.
6. Identify film abnormalities, given a history and x-ray film.
7. Use that information to adjust a physical therapy treatment program, given x-ray film abnormalities.

STANDARD VIEWS

The two standard views used to visualize the femoral head and neck from two directions are the anteroposterior view and the frog-leg view.

EVALUATION OF THE HIP USING ABCS

Anteroposterior View
Frog-Leg View

The AP view is taken with the patient supine and the hip internally rotated 15 degrees (Figure 6-1). The frog leg is taken with the patient supine, knees flexed, ankles together, and the femurs fully abducted (Figure 6-2). Its purpose is to give a second, lateral view of the proximal femur. This view is never used to rule out a fracture of the proximal femur or a dislocated hip since it places too much torque on the hip joint. If occult injuries are suspected, such as a fractured acetabulum, computed tomography (CT) in the axial plane or frontal plane is employed. What may appear as a questionable fracture line on x-ray will clearly be visible on CT.

Alignment

Points of alignment on an AP view of the hip and pelvis include:

1. Identify the major anatomical landmarks of the pelvis and proximal femurs. Note the following lines and points of identification:
   a. The **iliopubic** and **ilioischial** lines. These two lines represent the anterior and posterior columns of the pelvis respectively. The iliopubic line runs from the midpoint of the inner rim of the pelvis distally along the medial rim of the pelvis toward the pubic rami. The ilioischial line originates in the same place and runs distally along the medial border of the "teardrop" to the medial border of the obturator foramen.

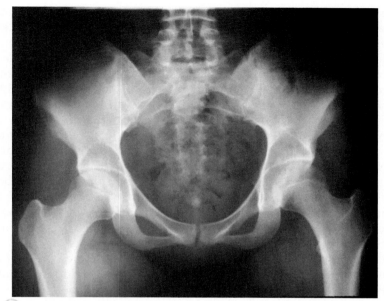

F*igure* 6-1. ■ **A standard AP view of the pelvis and hips.** Note the teardrops.

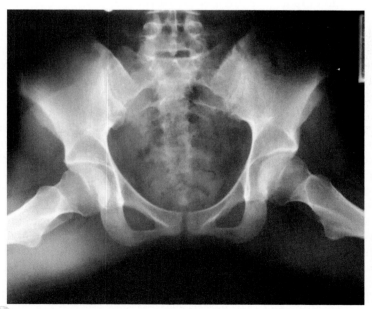

F*igure* 6-2. ■ **A standard frog-leg view of the hips.** Note how well the spherical shape of the femoral head is shown.

     b. **Teardrop(s)** represent(s) the sum of the shadows created by the acetabular walls. They should be equal distance from the medial pelvic rim and the femoral heads.

     c. **The center edge angle (of Wiberg)** is an angle created when a line is drawn from the center of the femoral head vertically and another is drawn from the same center point to the proximal, lateral edge of the acetabular rim. The angle formed must be greater than 25 degrees in an adult or dysplasia of the hip exists.

     d. **Shenton's line** is a line drawn from the medial edge of the proximal femur metaphysis proximally and medially along the proximal rim of the obturator foramen. Normally, this is a smooth line. If there is an offset or discontinuity in the line from its femoral metaphysis to the obturator edge, it may indicate a fracture, subluxation, or dislocation.

2. Evaluate the pelvis to determine if the iliac crests are level or if the entire pelvis is shifted or tilted in the coronal plane. If the pelvis is rotated, there will be accompanying shifts in the other alignment points.

3. Are the pubic rami aligned in the coronal plane? An AP view will not visualize the alignment of the pubic rami axial plane; this would require an "outlet" type view or can be evaluated via axial cuts in a CT of the pelvis.

4. Are the femurs equally rotated on this projection? The relative size and exposure of the lesser trochanters is an acceptable way of evaluating the rotation of the femurs.

5. Are the greater trochanters level at their proximal points? This evaluation point is valid only if the entire pelvis is level.

Bone Density

Density in the hip and pelvis varies by the type and view of the bone and depends upon understanding which bones overlap or superimpose over others on certain views. The margins of the acetabulum on AP films are "shadows," and recognition of these important shadows takes practice by knowing that, on the AP view of the hip and pelvis, the anterior rim is superior and medial to the posterior rim (Figure 6-3).[2] Increases in density of the pelvis may be the result of alignment, as in the overlay of the iliac wings with the sacrum posteriorly on the AP view or from more dynamic processes, such as sclerosis (thickening—seen on plain films as a "whitening" of the subchondral bone), resulting from bone-on-bone articulation when the hyaline-articular cartilage is damaged or worn. Other causes of increased density can result from insults to the bone or periosteum from a fracture or trauma. The increased density seen in the femoral neck from an overuse or repetitive stress injury manifests itself on plain films as a small area of increased density along the superior portion of the neck or inferior portion of the neck depending upon whether the insults are compressive or distractive. This is discussed further in the pathology portion of this chapter. An insult to the periosteum results in a nonspecific reaction by the periosteum. The periosteum lays down bone in a specific pattern that depends upon the type and duration of the pathologic condition. A slowly developing stress reaction may have time to demonstrate partial healing, typically seen

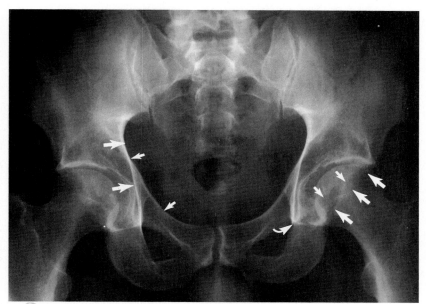

Figure 6-3. ■ Note *left to right:* the ischial line, iliopubic line, anterior rim of the acetabulum and posterior rim of acetabulum. *(From Manaster BJ: Adult chronic hip pain: radiographic evaluation,* Radiographics *20:S3-S25, 2000.)*

as a small area of increased density, whereas a rapidly growing tumor may show a more "hair-on-end" or "sunburst" pattern, as seen in an osteosarcoma (Figure 6-4).

The proximal portion of the femur develops strong trabecular patterns along the lines of compressive and distractive forces in accordance with Wolff's law. The four major trabecular patterns are: (1) principal compressive group, (2) secondary compressive group, (3) principal tensile group, and (4) secondary tensile group (Figure 6-5).[1]

The triangular space formed by the margins of the principal and secondary compressive trabeculae on an AP view of the proximal femur and bordered proximally by the principal tensile trabeculae is known as the "Ward's triangle.[1]"

Bone Dimension

The pelvis and the proximal femur offer the advantage that the two sides are visible simultaneously on the standard AP x-ray. The hip and pelvis are evaluated for symmetry throughout. Particular attention should be focused on the proximal femur. Following trauma, Shenton's line should be run bilaterally and the center edge angle measured to ensure that the femoral head maintains its normal relationship with the acetabulum. One side is always carefully compared with the opposite side (Figure 6-6).

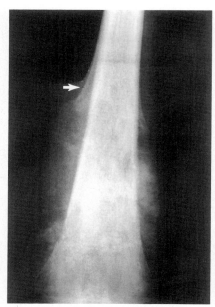

Figure 6-4. ■ **X-ray of osteosarcoma that demonstrates the characteristic sunburst pattern.** *(From Kumar V, Abbas AK, Fausto N:* Robbins and Cotran pathologic basis of disease, *ed 7 Philadelphia, 2005, Saunders.)*

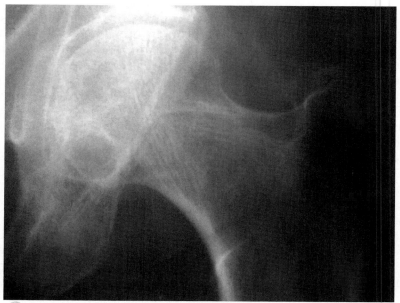

Figure 6-5. ■ This film demonstrates major trabecular patterns in the hip.

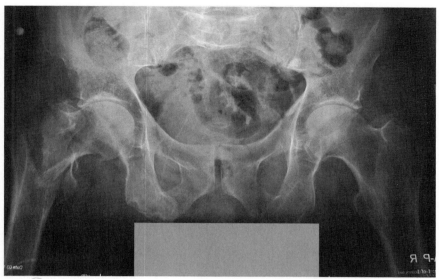

Figure 6-6. ■ X-ray showing changes in Shenton's line. Note the smooth curve on the right which represents Shenton's line. Compare it to the incongruent arc on the left where the arc of the femoral neck does not align with the arc of the inferior ischial curve.

The sacroiliac (SI) joints are compared left to right. Special attention is given to ensure that the iliac wings are both clearly visible and intact. On the AP view, the iliac wings run posterior to the sacrum, and osteolytic processes in either of these structures may not be identified immediately without specific attention to the separate margins of each of these osseous structures. The SI joints themselves are evaluated for symmetry. A marked unilateral change in the medial-lateral distance at the lateral margin of one of the SI joints may indicate swelling from an infectious process or pronounced ligamentous damage. An asymmetry of the SI joint after trauma mandates a careful evaluation of the pubic rami to check for an accompanying unilateral superior or inferior displacement or an increase in the distance between the bones of this joint (Figure 6-7).

The femoral neck and head require careful attention and analysis.

The pathologic conditions of the hip are grouped into categories that are very much age related. Skeletally mature adults do not develop Legg-Calvé-Perthes disease or slipped capital femoral epiphyses. Adults can develop avascular necrosis (AVN) of the hip from dislocations, prednisone use, trauma to the blood supply, and for occasionally unknown causes. In a healthy adult, the femoral head should be spherical shaped, particularly on the "frog-leg" views. The trabecular patterns in a healthy patient may not be as evident on the plain film x-ray.

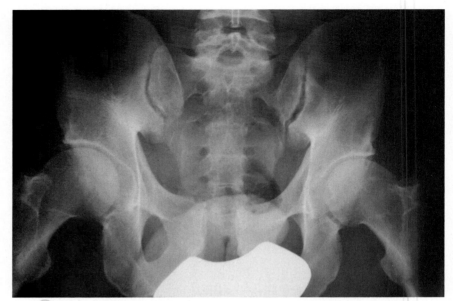

Figure 6-7. ■ This image is of a 30-year-old cowboy who had a large horse roll over his pelvis, resulting in a separated pubic ramus and SI joint.

Cartilage

Cartilage in the hip is of two types, the hyaline cartilage that lines the articular surfaces of the femoral head and the acetabulum and the fibrocartilage of the labrum that, much like the labrum of the shoulder, deepens and strengthens the hip socket. On an AP view of the hip, there should be equal and well-maintained space between the superior edge of the femoral head and the acetabulum. Decreased space on one side as compared with the other side is often an indication of early unilateral osteoarthritis (OA) (Figure 6-8). Osteophytes on the edge of the acetabulum or the femoral head are additional signs of degenerative changes (Figure 6-8). In the older patients, there may likely be demineralization or osteoporosis as evidenced by decreased density in the bone and more evident trabecular patterns. The patient's pain and/or lack of significant improvement with care are always the driving criteria for any intervention or further referral.

Soft Tissue

Soft tissue in the hip and pelvis consists of pelvic contents and the muscles to control the upper legs and the back. Calcifications in soft tissues are a result of dystrophic causes 95% to 98% of the time, and the remaining 2% to 5% are the result of chondrocalcinosis, metastatic, or tumoral calcifications, and very unlikely, osteosarcoma metastases.[3]

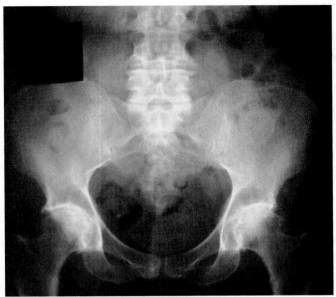

Figure 6-8. ■ **X-ray of OA.** Note decreased joint space bilaterally on weight-bearing surfaces, osteophytes, and increased density on the weight-bearing portion of the acetabula.

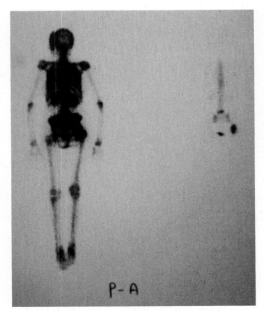

Figure 6-9. ■ Bone scan demonstrating positive reaction in the left hip; in this case from OA.

PATHOLOGY

Pathology of the Hip as It Relates to Chronological Age of the Patient

The radiology of the hip is normally the study of an inherently stable, weight-bearing joint where the pathologic conditions are strongly related to the age of the patient.

Congenitally Dislocated Hip

Some infants are born with chronically dislocating hips. The at-risk age group is birth to approximately 2 to 3 years of age. It is found in females more frequently than males at a 4 to 1 ratio. Eighty percent are unilateral (Figure 6-10).

Septic Hip

Septic hip is also a concern in this age group and older and is associated with systemic symptoms of fever, pain, and lab results indicating sepsis. These children usually limp and may have vague pain that they localize to the distal thigh and may be mistaken for knee complaints. This is an emergency problem that requires immediate physician care.

Legg-Calvé-Perthes Disease

Children from the ages of 3 to 12 years (average age at diagnosis is 7) are also at risk for Legg-Calvé-Perthes disease, a form of idiopathic, avascular necrosis that occurs in young boys more than girls at a ratio of 4 to 1 and in Caucasians more frequently than other races (Figure 6-11). The incidence is 1 in 1200.[4] Adolescents may have groin pain with activity or vague distal thigh pain.

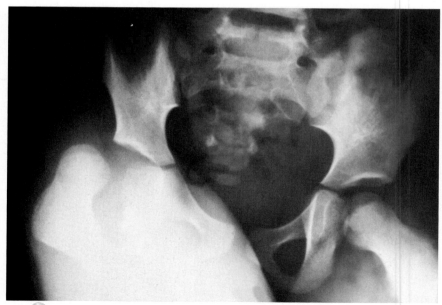

Figure 6-10. ■ Note that the right femoral head (left as we view the film) is clearly not contained within the acetabulum.

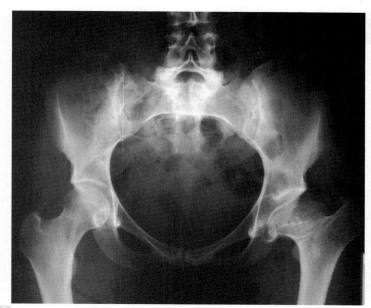

Figure **6-11.** ■ **Legg-Calvé-Perthes.** Note destruction of the right hip compared with the left, as a result of AVN. The right femoral head appears to be a melted ice cream cone.

Slipped Capital Femoral Epiphysis

Presentation of hip pain in the adolescent age group must also include in the differential diagnosis idiopathic slipped capital femoral epiphysis.[5] It is the most frequent cause of hip pain in this age group. Initially, it is seen on films as a subtle posterior-inferior movement of the capital epiphysis through the growth plate (Figure 6-12). This affects males only slightly more frequently than females. The British history of medicine in the United States lends itself to cultural and racial bias. The historical phenotype of the slipped capital femoral epiphysis was an overweight Caucasian male with immature genitalia. However, during the early 1980s in a large urban hospital in the southern United States, an adopted 14-year-old African male who was tall, slim, muscular, and genitally mature, but with x-ray evidence confirming bilateral slipped capital femoral epiphyses, was treated. We now know that this diagnosis is at least as common in African-American adolescents as in Caucasians.

Traumatic Hip Dislocation and Hip Fracture

Young adults are at risk for traumatic injuries from high speed–high risk sports involving motor vehicle accidents (MVAs) (Figures 6-13 and 6-14), large animals, team collision sports, skiing, snowboarding, etc.

Labral Tears and Acetabular Fracture

Some of these injuries in this age group are hip dislocations and labrum tears. Clinical manifestations of hip protrusion or shallow acetabula may also present themselves.

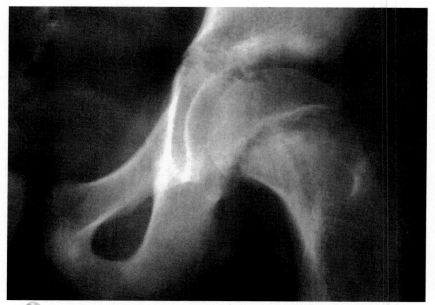

Figure 6-12. ■ **Note the increased distance on the growth plate and the distal migration of the femoral head inferiorly on medial side of the growth plate.** This patient has a slipped capital femoral epiphysis.

Osteoarthritis

Middle-age and older patients have problems related to OA or hyaline cartilage damage. Older patients, particularly those osteoporotic patients prone to falls as a result of inactivity or chronic balance challenges, are at high risk for fractures of the femoral neck. These may be subcapital, intertrochanteric, or subtrochanteric.

Middle-age and older adults often have diagnoses that relate to arthropathies, including OA; autoimmune diseases, such as rheumatoid arthritis (RA); and systemic pathologic conditions, such as osteoporosis. The hip is at risk for the usual age-related masses and tumors, whether they are malignant, benign, primary, or metastatic. Falls increase with age, and decreasing mineralization of osseous tissues results in increasing numbers of fractures of the proximal femur.

Alignment

Dislocations

Dislocations in infants are a result of congenitally shallow acetabula. Traumatic dislocations of the hip in adolescents and adults are the result of significant trauma involving falls, sports, and MVAs. The third category of interest to physical therapists is the postoperative patient following a total hip arthroplasty (THA). If a patient's postoperative intraspinal anesthetic is set too high or the highly medicated patient is not able to control their movements or the patient is

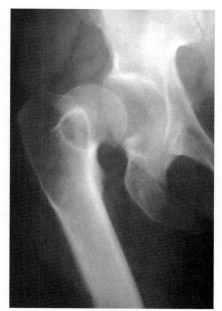

Figure 6-13. ■ This view is of a 23-year-old patient who sustained a posterior hip dislocation during an MVA.

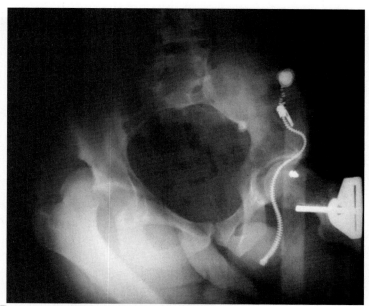

Figure 6-14. ■ AP view of a posterior superior hip dislocation sustained during an MVA. The zipper is from the EMS personnel's shock pants applied at the scene.

demented or disoriented, they occasionally remove the abductor pillows to prevent a fall when attempting to transfer onto or off of the bathroom or bedside commode. The posttraumatic injuries are not missed, but the postsurgical injuries may be unrecognized until the therapist does his or her evaluation before each treatment. Traumatic dislocations of the hip joint can be anterior, posterior, or central (medial) through the acetabulum. Traumatic dislocations may or may not have an accompanying fracture of the femoral head and/or the acetabulum. Only 13% of hip dislocations are anterior, and the majority are posterior.[6] Traumatic dislocations are normally diagnosed on the AP of the pelvis and hip, but a follow-up CT is indicated to rule out an occult acetabular or femoral head fracture. There are multiple classifications for the various types of hip dislocations and fracture dislocations, but most of the degrees of dislocation are tied to the location and type of fractures associated with the dislocation (Figures 6-15 and 6-16). Acetabular fractures can involve a fragment of the periphery of the hip or the central portion of the acetabulum (Figure 6-17).

Bone

Stress Fractures

It is not the purpose of this publication to review all the types of fractures of the pelvis and proximal femur and their prognoses. It is reasonable to explain that in a fracture of the femoral neck the more displacement of the proximal fragment relative to the distal portion of the femur, the less favorable the prognosis for healing.

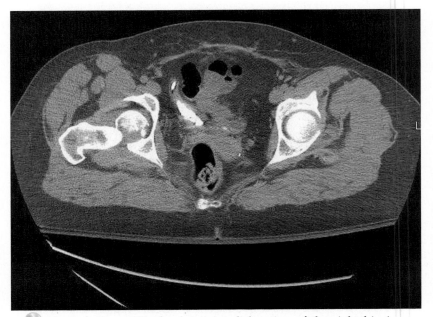

Figure 6-15. ■ CT of pelvis joint dislocation of the right hip in a 45-year-old female which occurred during a MVA.

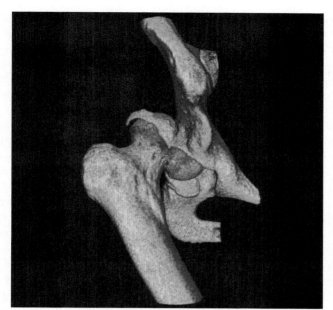

F*igure* 6-16. ■ CT of reduced right hip joint following dislocation in a 45-year-old female which occurred during an MVA.

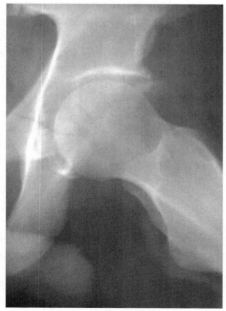

F*igure* 6-17. ■ Tomogram of the hip demonstrates an acetabular fracture.

Occult Fractures from Repetitive Stress and Pathologic Fractures. Fractures of the hip can be of the proximal femur or of the acetabulum. Review of the imaging is indicated for treatment planning or to assess the progress of healing when the patient is not progressing with their rehabilitation as expected or is experiencing increased pain. Those more likely to be seen in the physical therapy clinic, other than postoperative fractures, are occult fractures or stress fractures.

Occult fractures in the hip may be the result of low impact or repetitive impact injuries (stress fractures), and these may be referred to physical therapy as "groin pain or groin strains." Certain predisposing comorbidities, such as osteoporosis or abnormalities from metastatic lesions from prostate cancer, breast cancer, lung cancer, thyroid cancer, or renal cancer, are a few of the reasons for ongoing or worsening hip pain. It may be left to the therapist by default to determine the appropriate level of gait assistance a specific patient may require to protect the patient during rehabilitation if these comorbidities exist. Patients may be referred for "gait training" with a diagnosis of "metastatic disease" without accompanying imaging. This is a potential recipe for disaster. A patient with a metastatic lesion in the femoral neck is not a candidate for a cane, but requires the protection of crutches or a walker unless the referring physician is sure the bone is capable of tolerating the forces a single-limb stance (SLS) imposes upon the hip. To attempt to make this professional determination without access to appropriate imaging is truly "flying blind."

Review the femoral neck for evidence of increased or decreased density along the femoral neck (sclerosis or a lucent line). The incidence of these injuries is a function of the activity level of the population being studied. Several studies of track and field athletes indicated an incidence of 9% to 31%.[7] The range of femoral neck fractures was found in one study of 320 patients to be between 5% and 10%.[8] These injuries indicate compressive and distractive forces that the body is unable to accommodate quickly enough to prevent progressive weakening of the bone and eventual failure. Stress fractures are literally "slow motion fractures" until they reach the point of failure. The discomfort accompanying this process is normally self-limiting unless the individual is in a regimented training program. These stress reactions and/or fractures can occur in any weight-bearing bone undergoing undue repetitive stress, but are especially worrisome in the femoral neck. The physical therapist is uniquely suited to diagnose this pathologic condition. More frequently than one author would like to admit, patients have been referred to him with various diagnoses of "groin pull," "hip flexor strain," etc., when the actual diagnosis was an overuse or stress reaction of the hip.

This is a medical emergency, and the patient needs weight-bearing protection until imaging has definitively ruled out a stress reaction or fracture of the femoral neck.

The diagnosis is made initially by the patient's history. *Any patient*, regardless of age, who is involved in an "enforced" training regimen that involves weight-bearing repetitive stress is at risk. The enforced training regimen may be part of: military training, sports team competitive training at any level, or personal training, such as preparing for a marathon, mountain climbing expedition, or backpacking adventure. Snowdy et al in an article in the *American Journal of Sports Medicine* (AJSM) published in 1988 reported that the most reliable clinical symptom of an impending stress fracture of the hip is "groin pain" (Figures 6-18 and 6-19).[9] If the initial x-rays are negative, a bone scan may be indicated to rule out the diagnosis definitively. Remember that bone scans are nonspecific. They do not tell the clinician what is causing the increased metabolic activity in the bone, just that there is increased metabolic activity. There has been at least one case of a stress fracture of the hip in an active young male that was read as negative on the initial bone scan, but proved to be positive on a follow-up MRI 3 months after the bone scan. The patient had a release from his physician to resume running after the negative bone scan.[10] It is the clinician's careful history taking combined with careful physical examination and review of the available imaging that makes the physical therapy diagnosis. The patient may not be able be more specific than "groin pain" that is intensified with training. Extremes of passive motion may increase the patient's pain. Provocative tests, such as running on a treadmill or hopping in SLS, are risky in this diagnosis, and imaging before such testing is strongly recommended.

Osteonecrosis

Osteonecrosis, or AVN, as listed earlier, is a problem that can affect the femoral head in young children, adolescents, and adults. When viewing the plain x-ray films, a careful review of the femoral head is required (Figure 6-20).

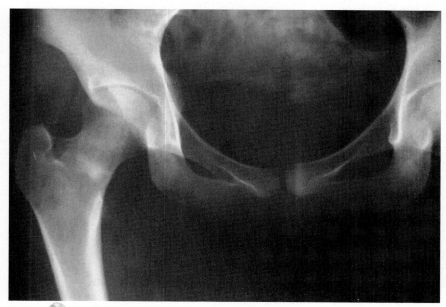

Figure 6-18. ■ This image demonstrates reactive bone formation perpendicular to compressed trabeculae on the right femoral neck.

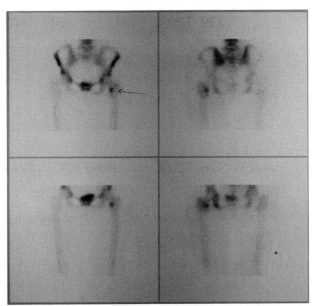

Figure 6-19. ■ **Image shows bone scans that are "hot," in this case from a stress reaction.** Other differential possible diagnoses include OA and tumor.

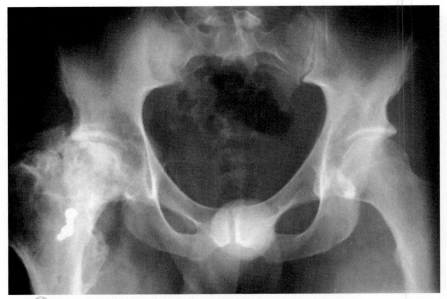

Figure 6-20. ■ **Tomogram showing increased density of the femoral head as seen in AVN.**

Often the first sign on plain films of osteonecrosis in young children is the increasing osteoporosis, but in adults it may be relative sclerosis in the femoral head and/or a "crescent sign," which is seen on the frog-leg view as a crescent-shaped radiolucency found along the superior medial edge of the femoral head.[2,6]

Cartilage

Pieces of labrum that may get into the joint following a dislocation can damage the avascular and aneural hyaline cartilage before the patient is aware of any pain. Femoroacetabular impingement is the result of: femoral retroversion, protrusio acetabuli, or coxa profunda. A cam type of impingement results from decreased "offset" between the femoral head and neck combined with retroversion of the femoral head, causing impingement of the anterolateral rim of the acetabulum and the labrum.[11]

At least one study indicates that early OA in the hip without a history of dysplasia is related to this type of impingement of the hip.[12]

Suspected impingement of the labrum is tested clinically with a test that positions the patient supine, and the involved hip is flexed greater than 90 degrees, adducted, and internally rotated using the lower leg as a fulcrum to internally rotate the hip. A positive test is accompanied by increased groin pain. If the patient is suspected of having a torn labrum, follow-up imaging is indicated.

Soft Tissue

Myositis Ossificans

Myositis ossificans, also known as heterotopic ossification, can occur posttraumatically in muscle or connective tissue.[12,13] It is usually visible on plain films within 2 to 4 weeks of injury. One type, "myositis ossificans circumscripta," usually encountered in contact sports results after a blow to the quadriceps, brachialis, or gastrocsoleus complex in an American football or soccer game. There is pain, swelling, and a mass in the region of the hematoma that presents the potential for loss of motion in the knee or hip. In some of these posttraumatic injuries, the patient may have experienced significant blood loss into the quadriceps muscle. Infrequently the patient may lose one or two units of blood into the region. Clinically, there is a hardening mass in the region of the intramuscular or intratendinous bleed. On plain films depending upon the length of time since the insult, usually 2 to 4 weeks, the mass appears to be partially ossified (Figure 6-21).

More importantly, in young athletes, this mass must be differentiated from an osteosarcoma or a soft tissue sarcoma, and no matter how comfortable the therapist may be, the final diagnosis must be made by an orthopedist or a fellowship-trained sports medicine physician. Myositis ossificans circumscripta on plain films is posttraumatic and calcifies from the periphery as opposed to an osteosarcoma that calcifies from the center of the lesion and "radiates" outward with the characteristic "sunburst" or "hair-on-end" pattern.

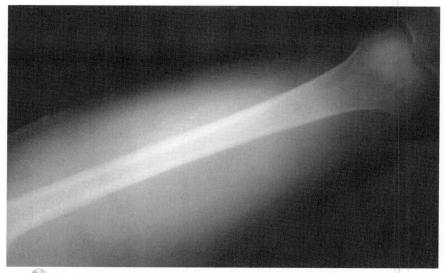

Figure **6-21.** ■ **Development of myositis ossificans.** Note the increased density above and in the physis of the femur in this 17-year-old male football player following a direct impact to his thigh.

Heterotopic ossification is usually found in the large joints of patients with cerebral or spinal cord trauma.

Soft tissue in the pelvis and hip, as in other areas of the body, may reveal swelling that can accompany:

a. Occult bleeding in the joint or surrounding soft tissues from fractures or sprains

b. Primary or metastatic tumors in the bone or surrounding soft tissues

c. Disease processes from drug use as occasionally found in AVN from legitimate and necessary use of prednisone for nephritis, asthma, RA, etc.

d. Trauma that results in dislocations with spontaneous relocation of the hip as found in MVAs, horse accidents, sports, etc.

CASE STUDY A

A 78-year-old female with a history of an infected total hip arthrotomy (THA) had a procedure to remove the infected prosthesis and to implant a spacer for the duration of the antibiotic treatment. In viewing the anterior-posterior film, is the spacer in the correct position?

AP Hip Spacer for Infected Prosthesis. Figure 6-22

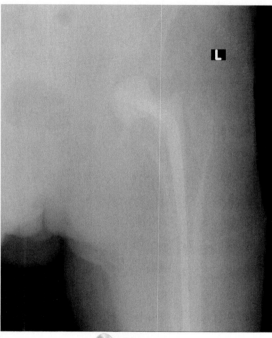

Answer: The spacer appears to be in the correct position on what is visible on this AP view. Note the distal portion of the prosthesis is not visualized. A projection including the opposite hip and/or a more lateral view—not a frog leg may be helpful.

Figure 6-22

CASE STUDY B

The patient is a 63-year-old male with a total hip arthrotomy (THA) who is now complaining of hip pain and inability to bear weight on the hip. Your Diagnosis? Plan of Rx?

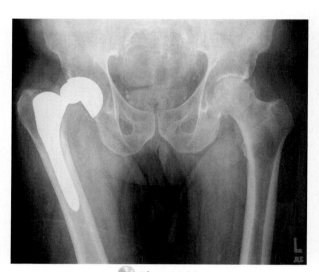

Figure 6-23

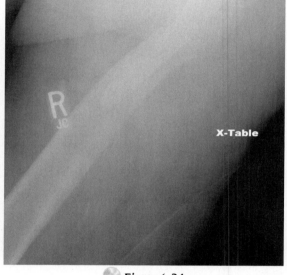

Figure 6-24

CASE STUDY C

A 12-year-old male was referred to physical therapy for evaluation and treatment of right thigh and knee pain. What do you see in the view of Figure 6-25?

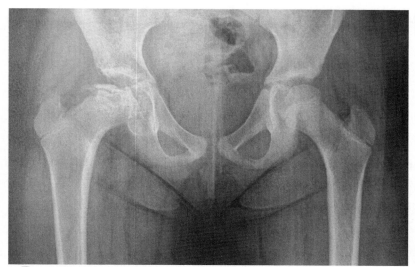

Figure 6-25. ■ This is not a hip study but the patient arrived with thigh and knee pain. These are MRI views. Remember that some children with Legg-Perthes' disease complain first of diffuse distal thigh pain and this results in an occasional short time of workup for knee pathology. © Kevin Shea, MD Boise, ID

REFERENCES

1. Rockwood CA, Green DP: *Fractures in adults,* vol 2, Philadelphia, 2001, Lippincott Williams & Wilkins.
2. Manaster BJ: Adult chronic hip pain: radiographic evaluation, *Radiographics* 20:S3-S25, 2000.
3. Richardson M: Approaches to differential diagnosis in musculoskeletal imaging. Soft tissue calcifications, The University of Washington. May 2008. Available at *www.rad.washington.edu.*
4. Nochmimson G: Legg-Calve-Perthes disease, *eMedicine* June 13, 2006. Available at *www.eMedicine.com.*
5. Loder RT: Radiologic decision making, Slipped capital femoral epiphysis, *Am Fam Physician* May 1988. 157(9):2135-42, 2148-50.
6. Greenspan A: *Orthopedic radiology*, Philadelphia, 1992, Raven Press.
7. Bennell KL, Brukner PD: Epidemiology and site specificity of stress fractures, *Clin Sports Med* 16:179-196, 1997.
8. Matheson GO et al: Stress fractures in athletes: case study of 320, *Am J Sports Med* 15:46-58, 1987.
9. Fullerton LR, Snowdy HA: Femoral neck stress fractures, *Am J Sports Med* 16(4):365-77, 1988.
10. Wen D, Propeck T, Singh A: Femoral neck stress injury with negative bone scan, *J Am Board Fam Pract* 16:170-174, 2003.
11. Clohisy JC, McClure JT: Treatment of anterior femoroacetabular impingement with combined hip arthroscopy and limited anterior decompression, *Iowa Orthop J* 25:164-170.
12. Ganz R et al: Clinical orthopaedics and related research, Femoroacetabular impingement: a cause for osteoarthritis of the hip. *Clin Orthop Relat* Res 417:112-120, 2003.
13. Person DA, Mandar A: Myositis ossificans, *eMedicine* pp 2-10, July 2006. Available at *www.eMedicine.com.*

7 The Knee

INTRODUCTION

Remarks

"The knee. The knee! Why is it always the knee?," lamented legendary American football coach Vincent Lombardi. It is a large, deceptively simple two-bone joint whose apparent simplicity belies the incredible complexity of its changing axes of rotation and the integrated neuromuscular coordination required for our species to perform amazing athletic and breathtaking artistic movements. Essentially, these athletic and artistic feats are performed on two sticks balanced end to end upon one another. The knee is located at the junction of the two longest bones of the body, the femur and the tibia, and these form the femoral tibial joint. This joint is one of two joints in the knee and consists of the cam-shaped distal femur and the very slightly concave proximal tibia with reinforcement from the ligaments and shock absorption and slight stability contributed by the menisci. The joint is subjected to enormous combined vertical, rotational, and tangential forces and is often injured by unanticipated external or repetitive forces. The anterior extensor strength and motor control of the joint is facilitated by a large sesamoid bone that creates the second joint of the knee, the patellofemoral joint. When healthy and properly aligned, this joint maintains the patella in the central superior-inferior axis of the femoral groove and distributes the large forces created by the quadriceps equally across the multiple facet surfaces of the patella. Dr. Steven Arnoczky's work with hyaline cartilage and synovial fluid has demonstrated how a healthy, well-aligned joint can dissipate the compressive and shear forces across the joint in an efficient manner.[1] The operative terms here are "healthy" and "well aligned." This chapter will discuss the knee and the information that can be gained from appropriate imaging studies of the knee.

OBJECTIVES ■

1. Recall the four standard knee views and their purposes.
2. Identify the normal and abnormal alignment of the knee.
3. Identify normal and abnormal densities of the knee.
4. Identify normal and abnormal cartilage on plain films.
5. Identify the normal and abnormal presentation of soft tissue.
6. Identify film abnormalities, given a history and x-ray film.
7. Use information from x-ray films to adjust a physical therapy treatment program.

STANDARD VIEWS

There are four typical views of the knee. The anteroposterior (Figure 7-1) (anterior-to-posterior or AP) and lateral (Figure 7-2) views visualize the knee as a whole from two directions that are at right angles to each other. The AP view demonstrates the varus-valgus alignment of the knee and the mineralization of the bones. Paradoxically the more evident the trabeculae the less the mineralization in the matrix of the bone. The AP view also demonstrates the medial and lateral alignment of the patella relative to the femur, osteophyte formation, and the maintenance of the joint space by the meniscal cartilage within the knee. The sunrise view (Figure 7-3), or variant thereof, such as the Hughston's and Knutsson views, is designed to visualize the patella in the groove between the femoral condyles. The tunnel or notch view is designed to show the intercondylar notch between the femoral condyles (Figure 7-4). The AP view is taken with the patient supine and the beam angled slightly—about 6 degrees cephalad. The lateral view is taken with the patient side lying and the knee flexed to 20 to 35 degrees.[2] If there has been trauma, a tunnel or "notch view" of the intercondylar notch with the AP beam directed to the knee at 40 to 50 degrees of flexion is helpful to visualize this region.

Figures 7-1 to 7-4 demonstrate the four views and how they are taken:

1. AP (see Figure 7-1)
2. Lateral (see Figure 7-2)
3. Sunrise (see Figure 7-3)
4. Tunnel (see Figure 7-4)

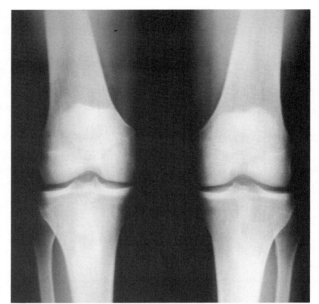

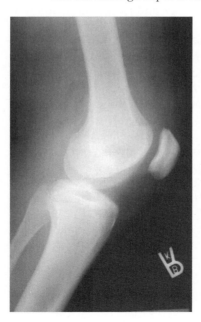

Figure 7-1. ■ **An AP view of both knees of a normal patient.** Note the alignment: the femur has a slight valgus alignment with the tibia, and the femoral condyles are congruent with the tibial plateau. The bones of the femur and tibia have smooth, consistent trabecular patterns. The articular surf aces of the femur and tibial plateau are smooth and rounded. The medial and lateral joint spaces are approximately equal, indicating that the cartilage depth is normal.

Figure 7-2. ■ **A lateral view of a normal knee.**

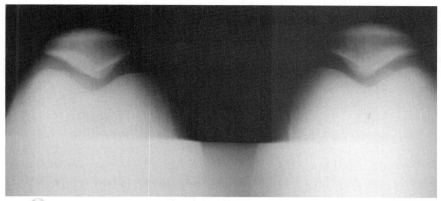

F*igure* 7-3. ■ A sunrise view of normal knees.

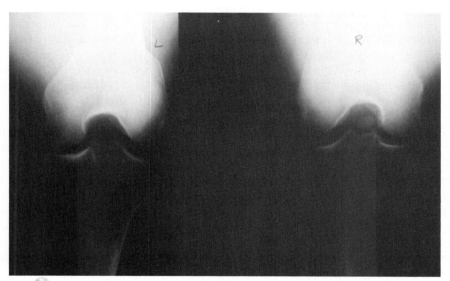

F*igure* 7-4. ■ A tunnel or notch view of the knees. Note the calcification in the notch on the right, indicating a cruciate ligament injury.

The ABCs system applies to each of the four typical views to systematically evaluate the knee. In this book, the structures that should be evaluated are labeled. There are videos of the evaluation process. The videos on the accompanying DVD may be accessed by going to the chapter on the DVD and clicking on the photo that you wish to see as a video.

ANATOMY; INCLUDING REGIONAL IDIOSYNCRASIES

The knee consists of two sets of joints, the patellofemoral joint and the tibio-femoral joint.

The patellofemoral joint is created by the articulation of the inferior surface of the patella and the intercondylar notch of the anterior, distal femur. It is a sesamoid bone that has developed in the distal quadriceps tendon to protect it from excessive shear forces as the quadriceps muscle contracts concentrically and eccentrically to extend and control flexion of the knee while the individual is weight bearing. It also provides the quadriceps an increased angle for leverage to facilitate knee extension. An accompanying result of this increased leverage is the significant increase in joint reaction forces generated in the patellofemoral joint during resisted extension and eccentric landing from a jump. The patella holds the quadriceps tendon anterior to the femoral condyles and anterior to the multiple axes of rotation about the joint, thereby increasing the extensor leverage of the quadriceps muscle. The marked extensor weakness exhibited by the quadriceps in a patient following a patellectomy is testimony to the mechanical effectiveness of this sesamoid bone. The patella is controlled by the quadriceps tendon proximally and the patellar ligament distally with medial and lateral support from the patellar retinaculum. The muscular alignment forces come primarily from the oblique vastus medialis. This muscle is the medial proximally aligned distal to portion of the vastus medialis muscle. It acts to oppose the laterally dislocating forces generated by the largest of the quadriceps muscles, the vastus lateralis.

Patellae come in various shapes. "Normal" or ideal patellar alignment is thought to be with the inferior surface of the patella equidistant from the surfaces of the distal anterior femoral groove with which it articulates. There is significant individual variability in the articular surface of the patella, as elucidated by Dr. Steven Arnoczky and Peter Torzilli.[1] The synovial fluid is non-Newtonian, and its viscosity decreases with increasing shear rate; the properties of hyaline cartilage and synovial fluid allow the healthy joint to tolerate enormous forces and repetitions with little ill effect.[1] Given the level of variability in patellar shapes and the depth of femoral intertrochlear grooves, the alignment of patellar articular surfaces is best likened to the keel of a boat that, when in motion and under load, floats or hydroplanes on the synovial fluid (see Figure 7-3).

Wiberg offered the first and simplest classification based upon the alignment of the inferior articular ridge relative to the joint.[3] Clearly, patellae come in multiple shapes as a result of an individual's genetic makeup and are then modified by the effects of the forces generated across the patellofemoral joint by the individual's skeletal alignment, muscular development, athletics, injuries, and work activities. Connective tissue plays an important part in the forces exerted across this joint. The articular cartilage on the inferior surface of the patella is the thickest of any articular surface and varies from 3 mm to 5.5 mm in a healthy young knee.

As a result of the high degree of variability in the shape and alignment of the hip, femur, and tibia, the patella may be subject to a variety of forces that may precipitate dislocation, subluxation, or wear and tear on the articular patellar surface. The results of these pathologic conditions may be visible on radiographs (Figures 7-5 to 7-10). Some examples of lesions detectable on plain radiographs are: osteophytosis, osteoporosis, bipartite patellae, soft tissue swelling, and mis-shaped and/or malaligned patellae. A marked decrease in the space between the inferior surface of the patella and the femoral intercondylar groove or notch indicates a loss of hyaline cartilage. Demineralized or overmineralized bone may indicate osteoporosis or systemic disease.

Tibia Femoral Joint

The tibiofemoral joint has the largest surface area of any joint in the body. It encounters extremely high forces generated by athletic activities, such as running and jumping, and work-generated forces, such as lifting from a squatting position. Damage to the ligaments and cartilage of the knee occur when the periarticular muscles—dynamic stabilizers—of the knee are unprepared for the trauma and stress, are fatigued and loaded beyond their physiologic tolerance, or when the ground is uneven and loading results in aberrant forces across the joint surface. When exterior forces, such as those experienced in skiing, soccer, or American football, exceed the capacity of the ligaments, they can fail. Alternatively, when repeated stresses weaken the ligaments over time, a relatively innocuous maneuver may result in a ligament failure, as in the

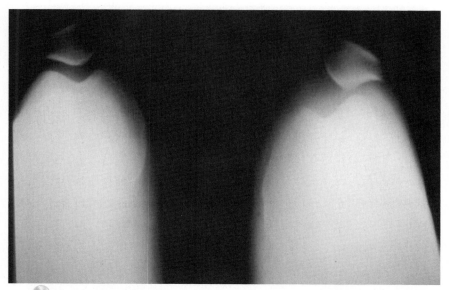

Figure 7-5. ■ **Sunrise view of both knees demonstrating a subluxation of the right patella.** Note that the patella has moved laterally and that the nadir of the patella is no longer aligned with the bottom of the femoral groove. Note that the patella *on the right* is riding laterally and at risk for subluxation.

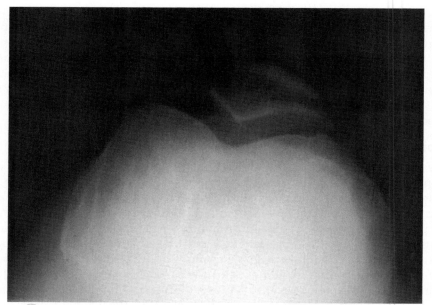

Figure 7-6. ■ Demineralized patella, osteophytes on lateral femoral condyle.

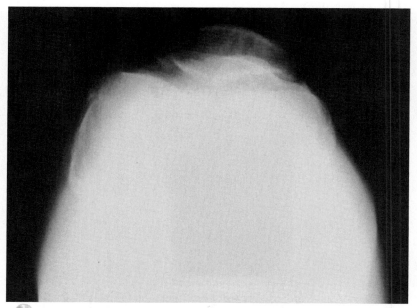

Figure 7-7. ■ **Sunrise view of the knee in a patient with severe arthritic changes to the retropatellar articular cartilage.** Compare the thick cartilage and clear joint space in the left knee in Figure 7-3 *(right side)* with this joint.

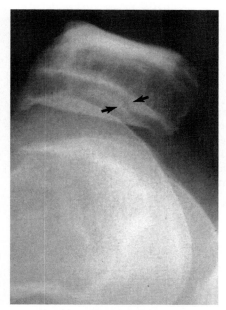

Figure 7-8. ■ Demineralized patella with oblique fracture.

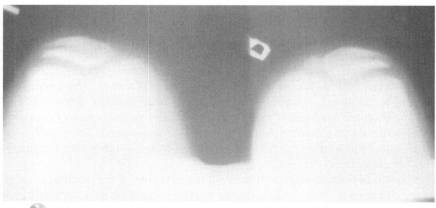

Figure 7-9. ■ Bilateral "jockey cap" patellae with bipartite patella.

noncontact rupture of the anterior cruciate ligament. Over time, nonphysiologic stresses on the knee will result in changes that may become visible on imaging. X-ray films give us a snapshot as to the current state of the knee, an additional piece of evidence to add to the history, examination, and laboratory studies to facilitate the treatment planning for the rehabilitation of the patient.

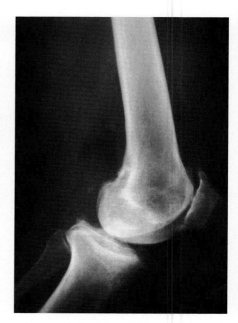

Figure 7-10. ■ **Lateral view of the knee demonstrating osteoarthritic changes to the knee.** Note the osteophyte at the superior and inferior poles of the patella and the osteophytes on the femur adjacent to the proximal patella. Also note the calcification in the tibiofemoral joint and in the posterior capsular area.

EVALUATION OF THE KNEE USING ABCS

Anteroposterior (AP) (see Figure 7-1)

Alignment

Normal Alignment. The normal knee when seen on an AP view will show a slight valgus alignment that varies by gender and individual skeletal alignment. The medial and lateral joint spaces will appear to be equal. The medial and lateral femoral condyles are slightly convex, centered, and aligned with the medial and lateral margins of the tibial plateau on AP views. The femoral condyles will be centered on their respective tibial articulations. The medial portions of both condyles should be smooth and show no evidence of erosion by the tibial eminences (attachments of the cruciate ligaments). The patella is visible and superimposed on the femoral condyles, but is notably less distinct than on the AP projection.

The lateral projection will demonstrate the margins of the femoral condyles. The medial condyle, because it is larger, will be seen to project distally beyond the lateral condyle. The condyles will be centered relative to the tibial plateau, and the margins of the articular surfaces should be carefully checked for any changes in the continuity of the bone that may indicate occult fractures, avulsions, or osteochondral defects (OCDs).

Abnormal Alignment. Unilateral degeneration as a result of a longstanding absence of the fibrocartilage of the menisci in the medial or lateral knee compartments may lead to a varus (loss of medial meniscus) or valgus (loss of lateral meniscus) deformity of the knee, as shown in Figure 7-11. The unilateral absence of the menisci leads to severe degeneration of the hyaline cartilage and

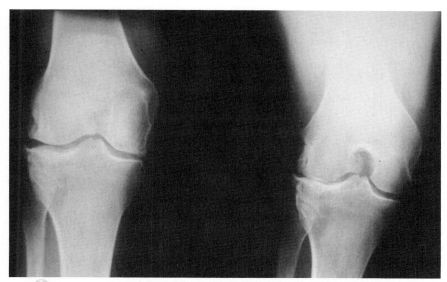

Figure 7-11. ■ AP views of two knees. While both views demonstrate flattening of the medial femoral condyles, *the view on the right* as we view this film shows a medial migration of the femur on the tibia and the impingement of the medial wall of the lateral condyle on the lateral intercondylar tubercle. There is also a complete loss of lateral joint space with resulting flattening of the lateral femoral and tibial articular surfaces and increasing density on the lateral tibial joint surface.

the characteristic "bone on bone" changes, including erosion of the surfaces and "whitening" or "eburnation" of the contact surfaces of the subchondral bone.

This malalignment ultimately leads to shifting of the femoral condyle medially or laterally in relation to the tibial plateau.

Bone

Normal Bone. The tibial plateau and femoral condyles are consistent cancellous bone with trabecular patterns aligned with the normal stress experienced by the bone. The cortical bone of the metaphysis and that portion of the diaphysis that is visible are smooth and without lucencies that may indicate occult fractures or periosteal reactions that may indicate stress reactions or tumors. As you trace the margins of the articular surfaces of the distal femur, they should be smooth and without breaks. The distal condyles are slightly convex to fit the concavity of the tibial plateau that is further enhanced and deepened by the shape of the menisci.

Abnormal bone. Several pathologic conditions may be seen in bone density or dimensions. OCDs may be visible on medial or lateral femoral condyles, as shown in Figures 7-13 and 7-14. Damage to the articular cartilage of the knee can be from an unexplained cause or abnormal loading of the joint surfaces. Damage to the subchondral bone may result in the formation of osteoarthritic changes to the joint surfaces. This articular damage when acute will result in significant,

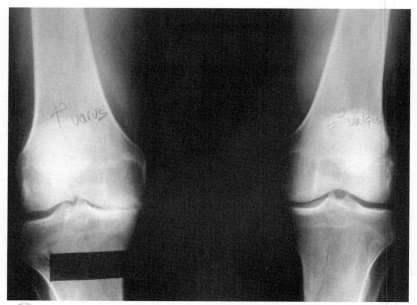

Figure 7-12. ■ **An AP view of a knee with degenerative changes to the medial compartment of the left knee.** Note the lack of joint space in the medial compartment of the knee on the left as we view this film. Also note the increased density of the subchondral bone about the medial compartment in an attempt to withstand the increased pressure on itself.

rapid intraarticular swelling since the subchondral bone bleeds rapidly and generously, and the synovium reacts to erythrocytes with the production of fluid exudates. This finding is cause for concern since articular chondrocytes have yet to demonstrate dependable regeneration (Figures 7-13 to 7-16).

Trauma or a loss of blood supply to subchondral bone may lead to an area of articular surface necrosis and falling away, leaving an articular defect, such as that seen in Figure 7-17. The portion that broke away may move about as an osteochondral fragment. The condition is known as osteochondritis dissecans (OD). The fragment may have to be surgically removed to prevent further articular damage.

Osgood-Schlatter disease is an inflammation which leads to partial avulsion of the insertion of the quadriceps ligament on the tibial tuberosity. It is somewhat self-limiting with skeletal maturation, but can be painful and significantly limit activities in the young student athlete (Figure 7-18).

A tibial plateau fracture may result from blunt or dynamic trauma (falls, sports, motor vehicle accidents, etc.) or when the bone is abnormally loaded with great force. Inordinate varus or valgus angulation of the knee in the absence of accompanying changes in the same side femoral condyle on the AP film mandates careful reexamination of the film for bleeding or other signs of

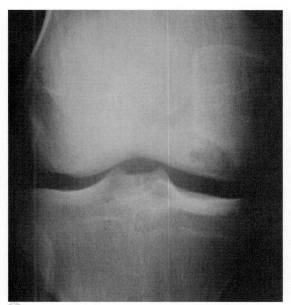

Figure 7-13 ■ AP tomogram of the medial femoral condyle of the knee demonstrating an osteochondral defect (OCD). Note the change in density along the condyle. *(Courtesy of Andrew Curran, MD Nampa, Idaho)*

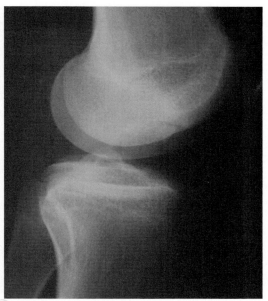

Figure 7-14 ■ Lateral view demonstrating an OCD on the lateral femoral condyle; note density change in bone. *(Courtesy of Andrew Curran, MD Nampa, Idaho)*

an occult fracture of the tibial plateau. Figure 7-19 demonstrates a mildly displaced plateau fracture. At first, the fracture may be subtle. However, if one follows the right margin of the proximal tibia, there is a slight incongruence of the border that demonstrates the fracture.

A patellar fracture may occur when it is "preloaded" by a powerful eccentric contraction of the quadriceps muscle as seen in a fall from a certain height or a unilateral landing—as in a rebound in basketball—especially if the patella is struck while under tension (see Figure 7-8). Patellar fractures are an infrequent but serious complication of one technique for anterior cruciate ligament reconstruction (ACLR).[4] The "bone tendon bone" (BTB) surgery harvests the middle third of the patellar tendon along with the attached distal, middle piece of the patella and a similar section from the insertion of the patellar tendon at the tibial tuberosity. A recent example of this occurred to the professional football receiver, Jerry Rice, who fell on the artificial surface of the football field with his recently reconstructed knee while catching a touchdown pass and fractured his patella on that side.

Note in Figure 7-20 that the surface along the apparent fracture line is irregular, suggesting a recent fracture. This must be differentiated from a bipartite or tripartite patella. If there is a transverse fracture in the patella, it will

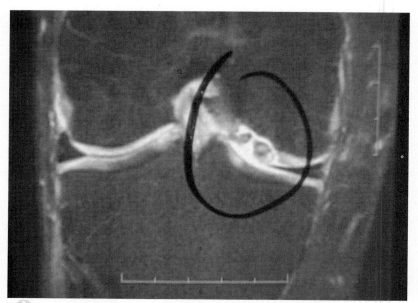

Figure 7-15. ■ MRI, coronal cut, T2, showing an OCD on the medial femoral condyle. *(Courtesy of Andrew Curran, MD Nampa, Idaho)*

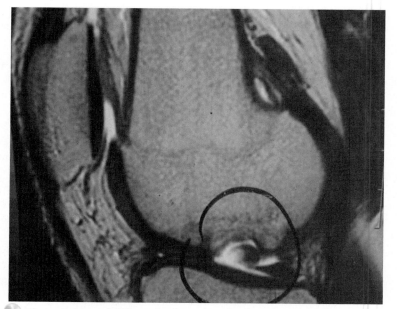

Figure 7-16. ■ MRI, sagittal cut, T1, demonstrating an OCD on the femoral condyle. *(Courtesy of Andrew Curran, MD Nampa, Idaho)*

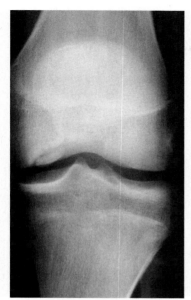

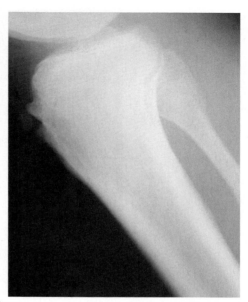

Figure 7-17. ■ AP view of the knee. As you follow the margin of the articular surface of the femoral condyles, note the *dark line on the left side* that connotes a separation of the articular cartilage from the femur. This defect, as it separates, becomes an osteochondral fragment or joint mouse.

Figure 7-18. ■ Lateral view of the proximal tibia. Note the bony fragment on the anterior proximal tibia. The explosive power of the quadriceps muscles begins to pull the patellar ligament away from its attachment on the tibial tuberosity.

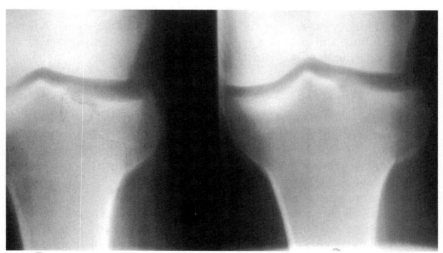

Figure 7-19. ■ AP tomogram demonstrating lateral tibial plateau fracture.

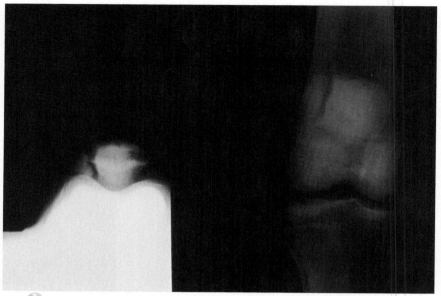

Figure 7-20. ■ A sunrise and AP view of a fractured patella. Both views reveal a fracture that separates the fracture from the main patella. Note that the fracture line is irregular in shape. The patella forms from three ossification centers, and some individuals fail to have the three bones united. They may have a bipartite or tripartite patella, which is normal for them. The edges of the patellar parts are smooth and consistent.

usually be visible. Without a history of trauma accompanied by significant swelling and pain, a patella with more than one component is most likely a "bipartite patella," which is failure to fully calcify the patella during normal development. In the case of the bipartite patella, the surface along the apparent fracture line is smooth.

Cartilage

Normal cartilage. When viewing Figure 7-1, there is a clear, wide joint space, representing the articular cartilage and fibrocartilage on the articular surfaces of the femoral condyles and tibial plateaus. The distal femoral condyles are smooth and rounded, and the subchondral bone is healthy appearing without increased density at the margins.

Abnormal cartilage. In Figure 7-12, note the diminished joint space of the medial compartment of the knee on the left. The appearance of bone on bone indicates an absence of menisci and that the articular cartilage has been completely eroded. There is bone-on-bone contact in the medial compartment, flattening of the medial femoral condyle and medial tibial plateau, and increased density in the bone.

Lateral View of the Knee on X-ray and Sagittal View on MRI

Alignment

Normal alignment. Figure 7-2 is a lateral view of a normal knee. The main alignment that can be seen on this view is the position of the patella. Is it high (patella alta), normal, or low (patella baja)? A general rule of thumb is that the length of the patella should approximate the length of the patellar ligament. The femoral condyles should align with the surface of the tibial plateau.

Abnormal alignment. The most obvious example of an abnormal alignment on the lateral x-ray of the knee is an AP dislocation of the knee as seen in Figure 7-21.

Patella alta, where the patellar ligament is longer than the length of the patella, is demonstrated in Figure 7-22.

Bone

Normal bone. In a normal knee, the margins of the distal femoral condyles should be smooth and congruent. The trabecular patterns should be consistent. Since the x-rays must penetrate both condyles, an increased density will be visible when the condyles are superimposed. The medial condyle is larger than the lateral condyle, and its distal margin extends more distally than that of the lateral condyle. Carefully examine or run the margins of the articular surfaces, the metaphysis, and the cortical bone of the diaphysis. The patella should show a consistent density and be without degenerative changes.

Abnormal bone. Osteoarthritis may be visible on a lateral view of the knee. Duncan and Saklatvala reported that three views, a weight-bearing posteroanterior (PA), a lateral, and a skyline view, will demonstrate 98% of the osteoar-

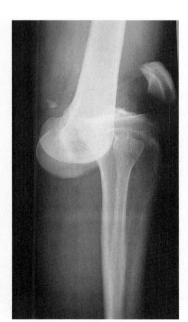

Figure 7-21. ■ Lateral view, demonstrating a posterior dislocation of the femur.

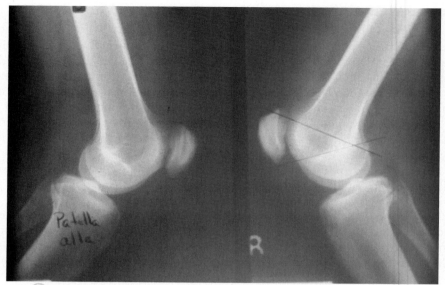

Figure 7-22. ■ **Lateral view of the knee showing a patient with patella alta.** As a general rule of thumb, the length of the patella should approximate the length of the patellar tendon. In this figure, note that the patellar tendon, which attaches to the distal pole of the patella and to the tibial tuberosity, is approximately 1½ times as long as the patella, indicating that the patella is riding high.

thritic changes in the knee in a clinically symptomatic population.[5] In Figure 7-26, we see an irregular surface of the patella with spurring. In this case as the knee extends, the patella rides above the lateral femoral condyle, which, along with the vastus medialis oblique (VMO) muscle, acts as a guide to maintain the patella in the patellar groove. The relative depth of the intercondylar groove is highly variable, as is the relative alignment of the patellae within this groove. The lack of bony control may contribute to the failure of the patella to track centrally. Certainly, there is some x-ray evidence to suggest that laterally tracking patellae undergo adaptive changes (Wolff's law) to accommodate variations in alignment.

The surface of the tibial plateau also shows an increased subchondral density and irregular surface area that is indicative of arthritic changes to the joint.

Osgood-Schlatter disease is seen in pubescent youth (see Figure 7-18). It is thought to be caused by a rapid increase in muscle strength of the quadriceps muscles that pull on the tibial tuberosity, which has not yet completely calcified its growth plate. The result is that the tibial tuberosity is pulled partially away or incompletely avulsed from the tibia, resulting in pain and a bony prominence just distal to the anterior knee. Note the light calcification in the area of

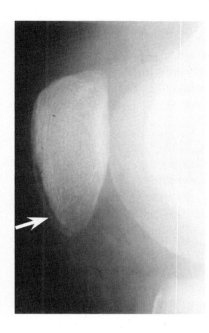

***Figure* 7-23.** ■ *(From DeLee JC, Drez D:* DeLee and Drez's Orthopaedic Sports Medicine, *ed 2, Saunders, Philadelphia, 2003.)*

the distal patellar ligament. This is evidence of the body's attempt to repair this traction injury.

A lucency at the distal pole of the patella is consistent with Larsen-Johansson disease (jumper's knee). This condition is similar to Osgood-Schlatter disease, except that the population is older and the growth plate of the tibial tuberosity has closed. Therefore in this condition, which usually occurs in young men in their 20s, development of explosive power in the quadriceps can generate more force than the patellar ligament can control. Microtearing at the insertion of the ligament to the distal patella causes the body to calcify the area in an attempt to strengthen the weakened area (Figure 7-23).

Stress fractures occur when bone is repetitively loaded without giving the bone time to increase its strength. Stress fractures occur when there is a rapid increase in bone loading over a short period of time. Typically, reactions are sufficiently painful to cause the participant to lower his or her activity levels and reverse the overloading. Stress fractures represent a failure of training, coaching, supervision, or, if the patient sought help, of the health care system to recognize the entity, seen where the individual pushes through (or is pushed through) his or her pain tolerance until the repetitive loading results in a fracture. Stress fractures are most commonly seen in military recruits and in highly competitive athletes in an enforced (self-imposed or coached) training regimen. An altered gait is usually evident before the evidence of bony changes on x-ray, and a bone scan will always demonstrate these changes before the plain film evidence.

Stress reactions and even early stress fractures are not usually visible on plain film x-rays because the bone is held in place by the periosteum and there is no angulation. Stress fractures usually begin 2 to 3 weeks after a rapid increase in activity. If these reactions are caught early, a 2-week period of decreased physical stress, or in the athlete's case, cross training without impact, with a slow resumption of regular activity will allow the bone to react in accordance with Wolff's law to strengthen and prevent the stress fracture. The key is to have the patient respect his or her pain as a warning sign and not exercise to the point of bone pain.

Typically a stress reaction or early fracture is not seen on x-ray film until we see the body's reaction to the fracture with resulting subperiosteal reaction and/or bone hypertrophy or evidence of an overt fracture line. Figure 7-24 shows a tibial stress fracture that progressed to a complete fracture and is now healing.

This plain film reveals the nature of the overuse-stress fracture syndrome, a fracture occurring in "slow motion" (Figure 7-25). The stress occurs in this situation from the posterior cortex of the proximal tibia and progresses anteriorly. The posterior cortex demonstrates a strong subperiosteal healing reaction with the deposition of a "healing callus," and the fracture line progresses anteriorly to the anterior cortex where there is not yet evidence of the fracture line through the cortex. This young athlete has clearly not heeded the body's message of pain in the proximal tibia and has continued to run and train on a fracturing tibia.

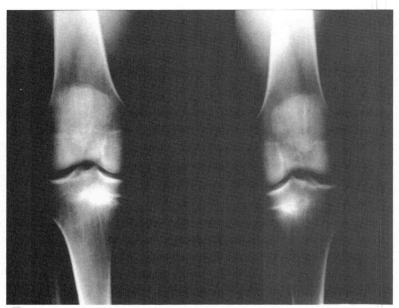

Figure **7-24. ■** Bilateral stress reactions of proximal medial tibias in a young female competitive runner.

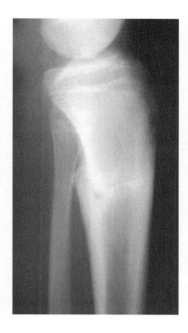

Figure 25. ■ **AP view of the proximal tibia demonstrating a fracture of the proximal tibia.** Trace the margins of the lateral tibia. A discontinuity is visible that represents a proximal tibial fracture. An increase in bone density about the fracture site demonstrates evidence of the beginning of bony healing of the injury.

Cartilage

Cartilage in the knee is hyaline cartilage and the fibrocartilage of the menisci. Tibiofemoral cartilage is evaluated on plain x-ray by a combination of checking for the maintenance of joint space on the AP view and lateral view and proper varus-valgus alignment. The lateral view is more sensitive for depicting OCDs since the medial condyle projects distally farther than the lateral condyle and allows an "edge" view of the distal femoral condyles.

The imaging of choice for cartilage and ligament pathologic conditions in the knee is magnetic resonance imaging (MRI). One arthrographic study of meniscal tears has shown that tears of the medial and lateral menisci usually involved the posterior horn of the meniscus.[6]

The following MRI images demonstrate several of the more common cartilage and ligamentous pathologic conditions in the knee.

On sagittal cuts running lateral to medial, the meniscus has a "doorstop" or wedge shape with the anterior and posterior portions of the menisci larger than the mid portions. A change in density in the substance of the meniscus is an indication of a tear. A truncated or blunt edge at the midsubstance of the anterior or posterior portion of the meniscus is another indication of a tear (Figure 7-26).

Normal cartilage. Normal cartilage is inferred by a smooth retropatellar surface that is not in apparent contact with the femoral condyles. Compare also the sunrise view shown later.

Abnormal cartilage. Diminished joint space between the patella and the femoral condyle is indicative of damaged retropatellar cartilage. Additionally, with loss of normal cartilage, there will be a subchondral retropatellar bone

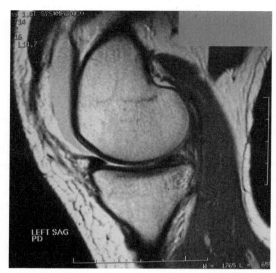

Figure 7-26. ■ MRI, sagittal cut, T1, demonstrates 'blunted' edge of the anterior portion of the wedge of the meniscus. *(Courtesy of Andrew Curran, MD Nampa, Idaho)*

response to abnormal pressure and friction with a resultant roughening of the retropatellar surface.

Osteochondritis dissecans. A loss of blood supply to the subchondral bone will precipitate necrosis and result in the sloughing of the affected region of the articular surface. This is sometimes visible on a lateral view of the knee along the lines of the articular margins of the knee joint. Fractures of the femoral condyles involve the distal 9 to 15 cm of the femur (Figure 7-27).[7] Note the missing area of articular cartilage in Figure 7-28.

Soft Tissue

Normal soft tissue. A lateral view of the knee does not usually show items of interest in the soft tissue. However, occasionally one can see a fabella in the posterior knee area, which may or may not be symptomatic. A fabella is a sesamoid bone in the lateral gastrocnemius muscle, which is present in approximately 10% of the population.

Abnormal soft tissue. It is often possible to see an osteochondral fragment in the knee joint where we should only see soft tissue. If the fragment is present, the patient should be further evaluated and additional imaging done to determine if surgical removal is necessary.

Although it is not present in normal films, with a lateral view of the knee, it is possible with a contrast dye to determine if a person has a Baker cyst. If a knee develops a chronic synovitis, the "jetting" of the synovial fluid pressure may result in the creation of a pouch in the posterior knee area that, most often under of the stress of athletic activities, results in popliteal swelling and a palpable lump. It becomes a reservoir that accumulates additional synovial fluid. Normally the

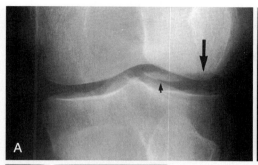
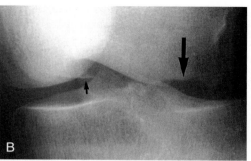
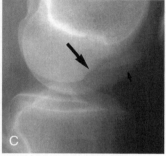

Figure 7-27. ■ AP **(A)** oblique **(B)** and lateral **(C)** views of the knee demonstrate a curvilinear defect in the lateral femoral condyle *(arrow)* representing an osteochondral injury and the displaced fragment *(small arrow)* located in the knee joint. Such injuries involve subchondral bone and the overlying cartilage, and are often the result of impaction forces. *(From Adam A:* Grainger and Allison's Diagnostic Radiology, *ed 5, Churchill Livingstone, 2008.)*

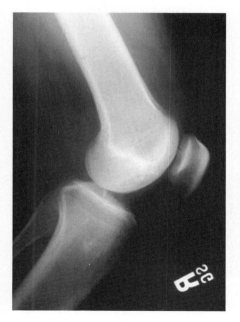

Figure 7-28. ■ **Lateral view of the knee showing an OCD of the femoral condyle.** This film initially looks normal. However, a close inspection of the articular surface of the femoral condyle midway between the patella and the anterior tibial plateau reveals irregularity in the articular cartilage.

lump resolves over a 2-week period until the next athletic activity. A Baker cyst can be demonstrated by an arthrogram. Radiopaque dye is injected into the knee joint, and the patient exercises until he or she experiences the full feeling in the posterior knee and a lateral x-ray is taken. The exercise is not always necessary. Dye in the area posterior to the tibiofemoral joint is seen below in Figures 7-29 and 7-30.

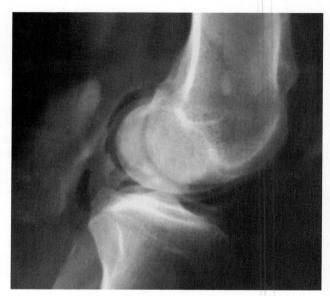

Figure 7-29. ■ Lateral view of an arthrogram of the knee demonstrating a Baker's cyst in the popliteal space. *(Courtesy of Andrew Curran MD, Nampa, Idaho)*

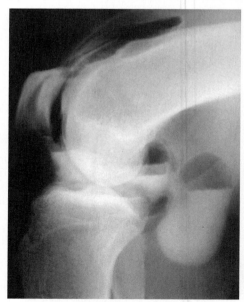

Figure 7-30. ■ AP view of the knee with a double contrast arthrogram. The knee was injected with a dye and with air to highlight the pouch posterior to the knee joint that has developed as a result of increased synovial fluid in the knee. If this pouch develops, it is called a Baker's cyst.

Sunrise View of Patella (To Visualize Patella on Femoral Condyles)

Alignment

Normal alignment. The sunrise view is designed to show the patella as it rests on the femoral condyles, as shown in Figure 7-3. Individuals have a wide variation in the depth of the intracondylar groove. Deeper grooves tend to hold the patella in a more normal, central alignment.

Abnormal alignment. The common alignment problem of the patella is a lateral subluxation, as shown in the right knee in Figure 7-5.

Bone

Normal bone. The undersurface of the patella should be smooth and congruent with the femoral condyles. Although the patella may show layers of different densities, they are consistent across the patella.

Abnormal bone. An irregular undersurface of the patella and/or femoral condyles is indicative of degenerative changes to the retropatellar joint, as shown in Figure 7-7.

Cartilage

To compare normal and pathologic views of retropatellar cartilage, compare Figures 7-3 and 7-5. Normal cartilage holds the patella well above the femoral condyles, and all bony surfaces have smooth surfaces. In comparison, damage to the cartilage results in arthritic changes to the subchondral bone in addition to the loss of joint space.

Soft Tissue

Soft tissue is not well visualized in the sunrise view.

Tunnel View of Knee

The purpose of the tunnel view is to visualize the intracondylar notch of the knee (see Figure 7-4).

Alignment

The femoral condyles should be in alignment with the surface of the tibial plateau. Joint space should be equal from side to side.

Bone

Bone density and dimensions of the tibia and femoral condyles are hard to evaluate with this view. However, these should be the only calcified structures seen. Other calcific structures in the film are either osteochondral fragments (joint mice) or possibly calcification of a partially torn ligament (see the right knee in Figure 7-4).

Cartilage

Although the cartilage of the knee is best evaluated with the AP view, in the tunnel view you can also determine if the joint spaces between the medial and lateral compartments of the knee are equal.

Soft Tissue

The tunnel view was not designed to visualize soft tissue. However, on occasion, a partially torn ligament may calcify and be visible with this view.

CASE STUDIES

CASE STUDY A

History: The patient is a 35-year-old male with a 2-week complaint of knee pain. He is physically active, but does not recall a specific injury to his knee. He began to notice pain in the knee with running and walking. He has a complaint of intermittent swelling of the knee.

Physical Findings: The affected knee is 1 inch greater in girth than the uninvolved knee. Full ROM is found. Quadriceps and hamstring strength is 5/5. Knee ligament tests are normal. McMurray's test and Apley compression tests are negative.

Imaging:

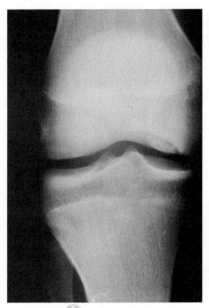

Figure 7-31

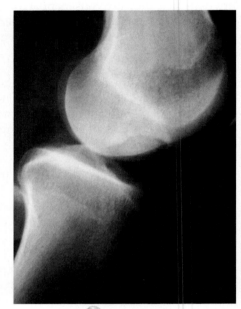

Figure 7-32

Image: Figure 7-31
Your impressions:
1. Alignment
2. Bone density and dimension
3. Cartilage
4. Soft tissue

Image: Figure 7-32
Your impressions:
1. Alignment
2. Bone density and dimension
3. Cartilage
4. Soft tissue

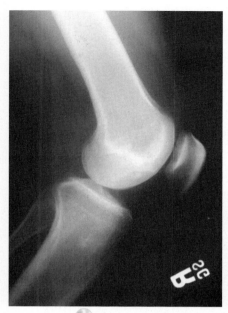

Figure 7-33

Image: Figure 7-33
Your impressions:
1. Alignment
2. Bone density and dimension
3. Cartilage
4. Soft tissue

Our impressions:
1. Alignment: Normal
2. Bone density and dimension: A lucency is noted in the articular surface of the distal medial femur consistent with OD.
3. Cartilage: Normal
4. Soft tissue: Normal

Therapy Questions:
A. What surgical treatments are available for this patient?
B. What would be your treatment?
C. What sports would you recommend and discourage?

CASE STUDY B

History: The patient is a 21-year-old male who injured his knee this morning while playing racquetball. He was weight bearing on his right knee when he made a quick cut to his left. He felt an immediate sharp pain in his right knee and was unable to continue the game.

Physical Findings: The patient is unwilling to bend and straighten the knee as a result of pain, and we are unable to assess muscle strength. The medial collateral ligament (MCL) and lateral collateral ligament (LCL) are intact. We are unable to assess the anterior cruciate ligament (ACL) and posterior cruciate ligament (PCL) because of patient guarding of movement.

Imaging:

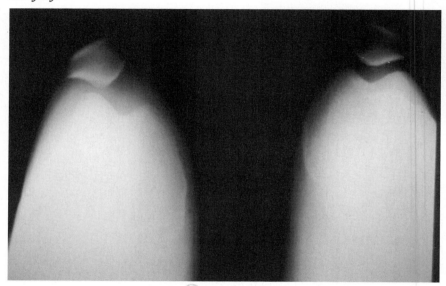

Figure 7-34

Image: Figure 7-34
Your impressions:
1. Alignment
2. Bone density and dimension
3. Cartilage
4. Soft tissue

Our impressions:
1. Alignment: The right patella is displaced laterally.
2. Bone density and dimension: Normal
3. Cartilage: Normal thickness
4. Soft tissue: Normal
   Subluxed right patella

Therapy Questions:
A. If you came upon this patient immediately after injury, how would you treat it?
B. What would be your treatment for the first 2 weeks?
C. What would be your treatment after 2 weeks?

CASE STUDY C

History: The patient is a 17-year-old high school athlete. Because of the heat, he had been doing his running at night. While running across the football field at night, he ran into a sprinkler head that struck him in the right anterior thigh. He developed a large bruise in the area. Now 3 weeks later, he is complaining of the inability to fully flex his knee and is having trouble walking.

Physical Findings (3 weeks following injury): The right anterior thigh remains swollen. The patient is unable to flex his right knee beyond 60 degrees. We are unable to test quadriceps strength because of the complaint of pain. Knee ligaments are stable. There is no complaint of knee pain.

Imaging:

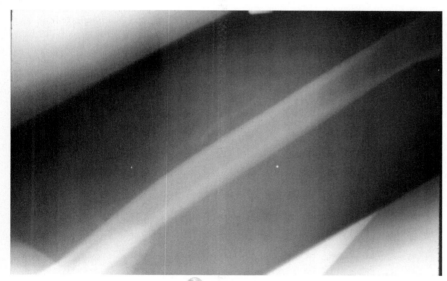

Figure 7-35

Image: Figure 7-35
Your impressions:
1. Alignment
2. Bone density and dimension
3. Cartilage
4. Soft tissue

Our impressions:

1. Alignment: Normal femur
2. Bone density and dimension: The margins and density of the femur are normal.
3. Cartilage: Not applicable
4. Soft tissue: There is an area of increased density in the quadriceps area consistent with myositis ossificans.

Therapy Questions:

A. What should be the initial treatment for this potential problem?
B. How aggressive should you be in regaining the lost knee flexion?
C. Are there any physical agents that may be useful for treatment?

REFERENCES

1. Arnoczky SP, Torzilli PA: The biology of cartilage in rehabilitation of the injured knee, In Hunter LY, Funk FJ, editors: St Louis, 1984, Mosby.
2. Resnick D, Niwayama G: Diagnosis of bone and joint disorders, ed 2, Philadelphia, 1998, Saunders.
3. Wiberg G: Roentgenographic and anatomic studies on the femoro-patellar joint, *Acta Orthop Scand* 12:319-410.
4. Johnson D: Graft choice for ACL reconstruction. International Society of Arthroscopy, Knee Surgery and Orthopaedic Sports Medicine, *Curr Concepts*.
5. Duncan RC, Saklatvala J, Croft PR: Prevalence of radiographic osteoarthritis—it all depends on your point of view. *Rheumatology (Oxford)* 45(6):757-60, 2006. Epub 2006.
6. DeSmet AA: Meniscal tears on knee arthrography: patterns of arthrographic abnormalities, *Skeletal Radiol* 14(14):280-285, 1985.
7. Tandeter H, Shvartzman P, Stevens M: Acute knee injuries: use of decision rules for selective radiograph ordering, *Am Fam Physician* Dec 1999.

8 | The Leg, Ankle, and Foot

INTRODUCTION

Remarks

The ankle and foot represent the interface between the bipedal body and the surface it contacts. It is a marvel of evolutionary adaptation and engineering design. The muscles of the foot control the toes, but the ankle is controlled by extrinsic muscles from the lower leg. These extrinsic muscles stabilize and power the ankle and foot, but stabilization of the ankle joint is assisted by the bones, ligaments, and tendons for control, balance, and shock dissipation during the various levels of gait and physical activity. The amount of force dissipation and shock absorption across the ankle and foot is remarkable. It is responsible for a large proportion of the imaging and x-rays performed in any emergency room.[1]

OBJECTIVES

1. Recall the three standard views of the leg and the foot and their purposes.
2. Identify normal and pathologic alignment of the standard views.
3. Identify normal and pathologic densities and dimensions of the leg, foot, and ankle.
4. Identify normal and pathologic cartilage.
5. Identify the normal and pathologic presentation of soft tissue.
6. Given a history and x-ray film, identify film abnormalities.
7. Given x-ray film abnormalities, use that information to adjust a physical therapy treatment program.

STANDARD VIEWS

The three standard x-ray views for the ankle are: the anteroposterior (AP) view, the lateral view, and the mortise view. The AP view projects through the body of the talus and the distal tibia, with the posterior tibial tubercle seen as an increased density in the mid portion of the proximal talus (Figure 8-1). The inferior, medial portion of the tibia overlays the distal fibula. In the AP view, the ankle joint is oriented with 15 to 20 degrees of external rotation relative to the coronal plane of the knee. To examine the entire joint without overlay from the fibula, the mortise view is added to the standard AP and lateral views. The lateral view (Figure 8-2) demonstrates the plafond (distal articular surface of the tibia) and the talus; the posterior tibial tubercle, or "malleolus" of the distal tibia; and an excellent lateral view of the calcaneus and the tarsal bones. The mortise view (Figure 8-3) is essential to fully visualize the relationship between the talus and the plafond and is required for a complete evaluation of the ankle joint.

Now evaluate Figures 8-4 and 8-5 using the ABCS to search for abnormal findings. Note that the AP view in Figure 8-4 appears normal until we see the fracture of the tibia in the mortise view. Likewise, the lateral view in Figure 8-5 appears normal, whereas the mortise view clearly demonstrates a fracture.

Special views include medial and lateral obliques. The medial oblique demonstrates the sinus tarsi, or tarsal canal, and the neck of the talus (Figure 8-6). The lateral oblique (Figure 8-7) may be helpful to evaluate a patient recently injured to rule out damage to the malleoli.

In the case of the patient with little or no trauma but significant ankle pain that may be refractory to conservative management, imaging is indicated, and

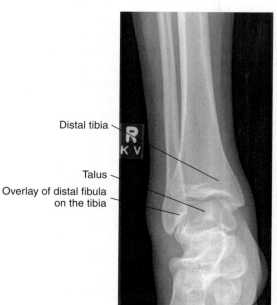

Distal tibia

Talus

Overlay of distal fibula
on the tibia

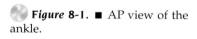
Figure 8-1. ■ AP view of the ankle.

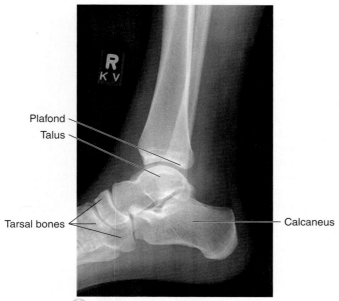

Plafond

Talus

Tarsal bones

Calcaneus

Figure 8-2. ■ Lateral view of the ankle.

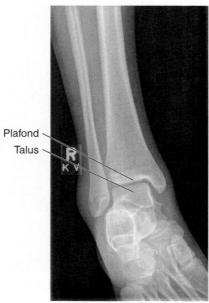

Plafond

Talus

Figure 8-3. ■ Mortise view of the ankle.

AP view   Mortise

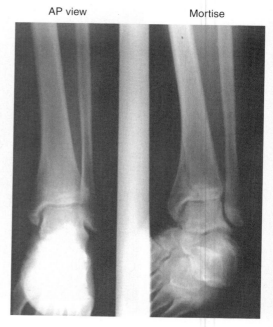

Figure 8-4. ■ **Demonstrates non-displaced intraarticular tibial fracture of the distal tibia.** Figures 8-4 and 8-5 show two views, side by side, a mortise and a lateral and a mortise and an AP, in which the lateral and the AP appear normal, and the mortise clearly demonstrates the fracture.

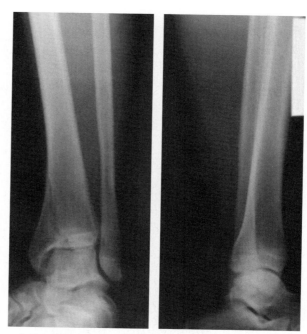

Figure 8-5. ■ **Demonstrates nondisplaced intraarticular tibial fracture of the distal tibia.** Figures 8-4 and 8-5 show two views, side by side, a mortise and a lateral and a mortise and an AP, in which the lateral and the AP appear normal, and the mortise clearly demonstrates the fracture.

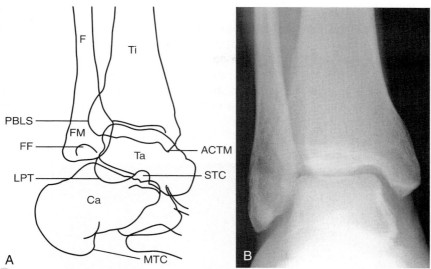

Figure 8-6. ■ **Medial oblique ankle view.** This view will occasionally demonstrate a fracture on the malleoli that is not visible on the three standard views. ACTM, anterior colliculus (of tibial malleolus); Ca, calcaneus; F, fibula; FF, fibular (digital) fossa; FM, fibular malleolus; LPT, lateral process (talus); MTC, medial tuberosity (aka medial tubercle); PBLS, posterior border of distal tibial lateral surface; STC, sinus tarsi/tarsal canal; Ta, talus; Ti, tibia. *(From Christman RA: Foot and ankle radiology, London, 2003, Churchill Livingstone.)*

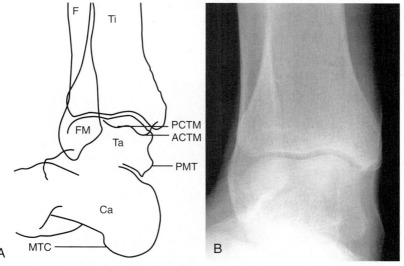

Figure 8-7. ■ **Lateral oblique ankle view.** May demonstrate a malleolar fracture not visible on the standard view. ACTM, anterior colliculus (of tibial malleolus); Ca, calcaneus; F, fibula; FM, fibular malleolus; MTC, medial tuberosity (aka medial tubercle); PCTM, posterior colliculus (of tibial malleolus); PMT, posteromedial tubercle (talus); Ta, talus; Ti, tibia. *(From Christman RA: Foot and ankle radiology, London, 2003, Churchill Livingstone.)*

comparison views can often be helpful to differentiate what is "normal" for this patient and what indicates a pathologic condition. If instability is found on exam or suspected, stress views or magnetic resonance imaging (MRI) may be indicated.

The standard views for the foot are: the AP, medial oblique and lateral. The medial oblique offers the best visualization of the articulation of the midfoot and forefoot. The lateral (Figures 8-8 and 8-9) and AP (Figure 8-10) views are necessary for the assessment of the toes.[2]

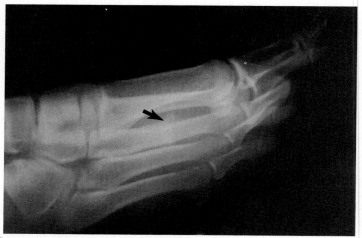

Figure 8-8. ■ Lateral oblique projection of toes showing stress fracture of third metatarsal.

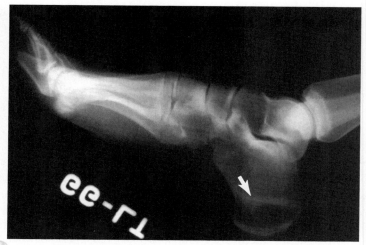

Figure 8-9. ■ Lateral of the foot, demonstrates calcaneal stress fracture.

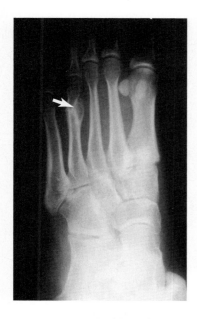

Figure **8-10.** ■ AP projection of the foot demonstrating a stress fracture of the fourth metatarsal.

EVALUATION OF THE LEG, ANKLE, AND FOOT USING ABCS

Alignment

The AP of the ankle view, as seen in Figure 8-11 *(left),* is evaluated for normal relationships between the distal tibia, fibula, and the talus. The bone surfaces should be smooth and equidistant from each other, except where the distal fibula overlays the distal lateral tibia. The posterior projection of the distal tibia (tubercle) should project clearly inferiorly to the superior surface of the talus.

The mortise joint is seen in Figure 8-11 *(right).* Alignment in the ankle is the relationship between the plafond, or distal articular surface of the tibia, including the medial malleolus, the articular surface of the talus, and the lateral relationship between the talus and the distal-medial fibula. The superior surface of the talus bears the weight from the plafond and dissipates or transfers the weight through the other bones of the ankle and foot via its articulations with the calcaneus and the navicular bone. It is critical to understand that the superior surface of the talus is not dome shaped, as it appears on the lateral view of the ankle, but is a spindle-shaped bone that articulates intimately with the plafond and that only a slight displacement of this relationship—as the result of the disruption of the mortise joint by a spread of the fibula from a fracture or severe sprain—may result in a shift of the plafond on the talus that disrupts weight bearing and/or causes the onset of osteochondral damage. A shift of 1 mm in the plafond-talus alignment reduces the surface-to-surface contact between these joints by 47%, markedly increasing the rate of wear on the osteochondral surface.[3] On the AP and mortise views, there should be equal distance between the superior surface of the talus and the plafond (distal articular surface) of the tibia. This space should be carefully traced from the medial to the lateral side. The superior portion of the talus should be centered between the medial and lateral malleoli on

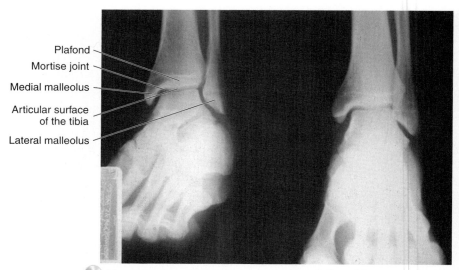

Plafond
Mortise joint
Medial malleolus
Articular surface of the tibia
Lateral malleolus

Figure 8-11. ■ Mortise and AP views of the ankle.

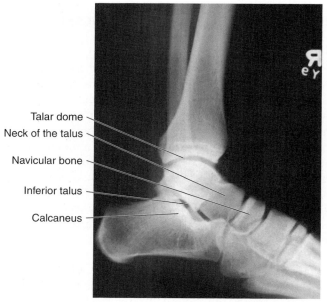

Talar dome
Neck of the talus
Navicular bone
Inferior talus
Calcaneus

Figure 8-12. ■ Lateral view of ankle demonstrating normal alignment, bone, cartilage, and soft tissue.

the mortise view. The fibula should be evaluated to ensure that there are no changes in its relationship to the talus. Also review Figures 8-1 through 8-3.

The lateral view (Figure 8-12) projects the superior articular surface of the talus as a dome shape, and on this view, there should be smooth, equal space between the articular surfaces. The neck of the talus should align with the na-

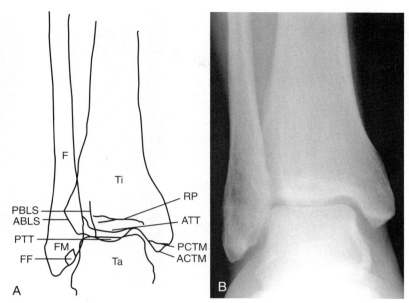

Figure 8-13. ■ AP ankle view. Note the overlap of the fibula and tibia in part B. ABLS, anterior border of distal tibial lateral surface; ACTM, anterior colliculus (of tibial malleolus); ATT, anterior tibial tubercle; F, fibula; FF, fibular (digital) fossa; FM, fibular malleolus; PBLS, posterior border of distal tibial lateral surface; PCTM, posterior colliculus (of tibial malleolus); PTT, posterior tibial tubercle; RP, remnant of physis; Ta, talus; Ti, tibia. *(From Christman RA:* Foot and ankle radiology, *London, 2003, Churchill Livingstone.)*

vicular bone and the inferior talus with the calcaneus, and the joint spaces should be smooth and equidistant.

The following drawings demonstrate normal x-ray image alignment: Figures 8-13, 8-14, and 8-15.

Bone Density and Dimension

The bones on all views should project appropriate density and healthy trabecular patterns that are oriented appropriately to the lines of stress across the bones.

The talus is the "keystone" of the ankle joint and is at the pivot point, or center, of the rest of the ankle and foot bones.[4] It is surrounded by the distal tibia superiorly and posteriorly (the third or posterior malleolus; think trimalleolar fracture), medially by the medial malleolus, laterally by the distal fibula, inferiorly by the calcaneus, and the navicular bone anteriorly. These bones are securely held in position and lashed to the talus by a series of powerful ligaments. These are divided into a lateral ligamentous complex and a medial complex. The talus is evaluated for areas of decreased density on the three views that may indicate fractures, particularly through the neck and/or through the body of the talus. If the talus is fractured, the vascular supply to the talus is at risk because the body of the talus receives blood flow from the superior portion of the bone, mandating follow-up even after the fracture is healed to identify avascular necrosis, if it occurs.

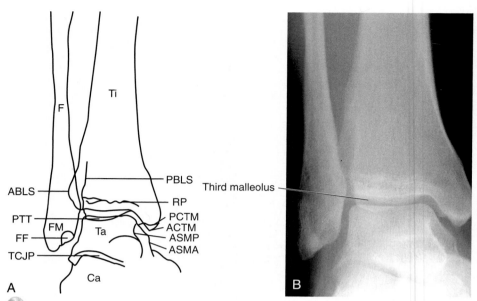

Figure 8-14. ■ Mortise ankle view. Note the equal distance between the plafond and the talus in part B. ABLS, anterior border of distal tibial lateral surface; ACTM, anterior colliculus (of tibial malleolus); ASMA, articular surface for medial malleolus, anterior margin; ASMP, articular surface for medial malleolus, posterior margin; Ca, calcaneus; F, fibula; FF, fibular (digital) fossa; FM, fibular malleolus; PBLS, posterior border of distal tibial lateral surface; PCTM, posterior colliculus (of tibial malleolus); PTT, posterior tibial tubercle; RP, remnant of physis; Ta, talus; TCJP, talocalcaneal joint—posterior; Ti, tibia. *(From Christman RA:* Foot and ankle radiology, *London, 2003, Churchill Livingstone.)*

Tarsal coalition (Figure 8-16) is a condition in which there is a union of the bones in the hindfoot, talus, and calcaneus or the midfoot, calcaneus, and navicular bone. This can be congenital or the result of trauma, infection, or surgery, and the coalitions can be complete or incomplete unions. If the condition is not obvious on the standard x-ray films, the computed tomography (CT) will give the definitive answer.

Cartilage

Cartilage evaluation in the ankle is directed to the hyaline cartilage between the superior surface of the talus and the plafond of the distal tibia. The joint should be carefully examined on the AP, mortise, and lateral views for any indications of decreased density. The anterolateral and posteromedial joints should be carefully checked for any subtle changes in density that may indicate osteochondral defects.

Soft Tissue

The importance of the connective tissue to the integrity of the foot and ankle cannot be overstressed. The ankle is so frequently injured in sports and active athletic pursuits that once a bony pathologic condition is ruled out by imaging

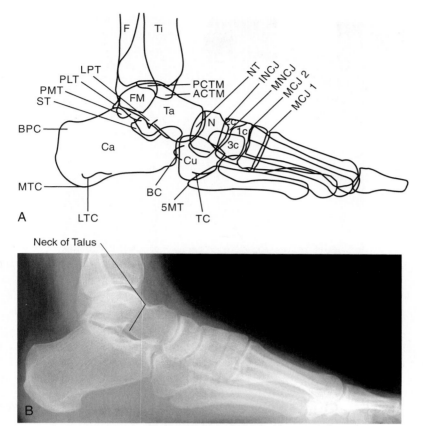

Figure 8-15 ■ Lateral foot view. Note the trabecular patterns in the calcaneus (stress fractures orient perpendicular to these) and neck of talus in part B. 1C, first cuneiform (aka medial cuneiform); 2C, second cuneiform (aka intermediate cuneiform); 3C, third cuneiform (aka lateral cuneiform); 5MT, tuberosity of fifth metatarsal base; ACTM, anterior colliculus (of tibial malleolus); BC, beak of cuboid; BPC, bursal projection, posterior calcaneus; C, crista (aka crest of metatarsal head); Ca, calcaneus; Cu, cuboid; F, fibula; LPT, lateral process (talus); LTC, lateral tuberosity (aka lateral tubercle); MCJ1, first metatarsal-cuneiform joint; MCJ2, second metatarsal-cuneiform joint; MCJI, interior aspect of first metatarsal cuneiform joint; MCNJ, medial cuneiform-navicular joint; MTC, medial tuberosity (aka medial tubercle); N, navicular; PCTM, posterior colliculus (of tibial malleolus); PLT, posterolateral tubercle (talus) (aka trigonal process); PMT, posteromedial tubercle (talus); T, (talus); TC, tuberosity of cuboid; Ti, tibia. (*From Christman RA:* Foot and ankle radiology, *London, 2003, Churchill Livingstone.*)

it mandates a careful "hands-on" clinical examination to localize the area(s) of damage. There is very little contractile and/or soft tissue on or about the ankle joint other than the ligamentous complexes. The muscles that do exist lend themselves to functional fine adjustments rather than major shock absorption or propulsion. The lateral and medial ligamentous complexes bind the joint together, and when clinical examination indicates, connective tissue stress im-

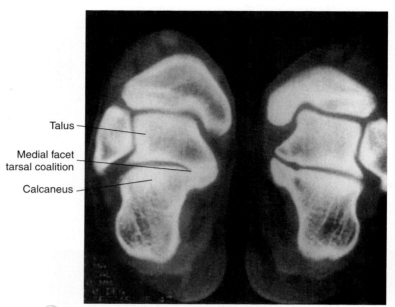

Talus
Medial facet
tarsal coalition
Calcaneus

Figure 8-16. ■ CT scan showing medial facet tarsal coalition of calcaneus and talus in young patient with frequent ankle sprains. (*From Canale ST:* Campbell's operative orthopedics, *ed 10, St Louis, 2003, Mosby.*)

aging is indicated with special attention to areas that reveal themselves as specifically tender during the clinical examination.

Soft tissue injuries in the ankle are injuries to the connective tissue and/or ligaments and osteochondral defects on the talus.[5]

The talus is supported medially by the medial malleolus and laterally by the lateral malleolus. These two struts are held in place yet allowed the required movement throughout the talar range of motion by: the medial ligamentous complex (the deltoid ligament complex); the lateral complex, including the calcaneal fibular ligament (CFL); the anterior talofibular ligament (ATFL); the posterior talofibular ligament (PTFL); the anterior inferior tibiofibular ligament (AITL); the posterior inferior tibiofibular ligament (PITL); the interosseous ligament (IL); and the interosseous membrane.[6]

The measurements for assessing the syndesmosis for injury on the three basic views of the ankle follow a "four, five, ten" rule. The first two measurements are on the AP view (see Figure 8-1). The first distance, not to exceed 4 mm measured on the mortise view (see Figure 8-3), is the distance between the medial edge of the talus and the medial border of the medial malleolus. The second of these is the horizontal distance, not greater than 5 mm, between the lateral border of the posterior tibial malleolus and the medial border of the lateral malleolus, also called the "clear space." The third is the tibiofibular overlap, not less than 10 mm, of the medial border of the fibula and the lateral border of the anterior tibial prominence. In the presence of normal measure-

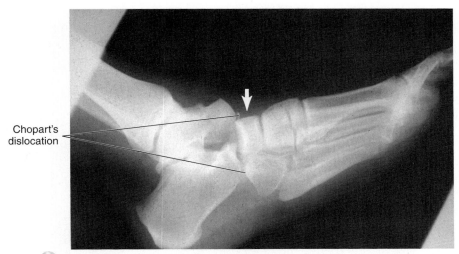

Chopart's
dislocation

Figure 8-17. ■ Demonstrates a Chopart's dislocation of the rear or hindfoot and the midfoot.

ments on the three standard x-rays, a symptomatic patient should be evaluated by MRI for evidence of tearing of the ligaments.[7]

PATHOLOGY

Alignment

Obvious malalignment of the bones of the ankle or foot without fracture can be diagnosed with plain x-rays. Further definition is provided with MRI to detect swelling of the soft tissues or bone marrow edema (BME). Study Figures 8-17, 8-18, and 8-19 before reading the legends.

Bone

The talus is the second most often injured bone in the foot after the calcaneus, and the neck of the talus is the site in the talus that is most frequently fractured.

The stress fracture or overuse injury in the fifth metatarsal is called a Jones fracture and is not to be confused with a styloid fracture, or dancer's fracture. A Jones fracture is a transverse (perpendicular) fracture of the proximal shaft of the fifth metatarsal. It can occur acutely by stepping off of a curb or as a result of overuse. The styloid, or dancer's, fracture is an acute avulsion of the styloid of the fifth metatarsal at the insertion of the peroneus brevis tendon. Both can be accompanied by a "pop" and result in immediate pain and swelling. The styloid fracture will heal well and at times requires only supportive measures, such as tape strapping, a walking boot, or a short leg cast, whereas a Jones fracture will need to be stabilized by an orthopedic surgeon with an intermedullary screw and, at times, bone grafting if it is to heal properly and not

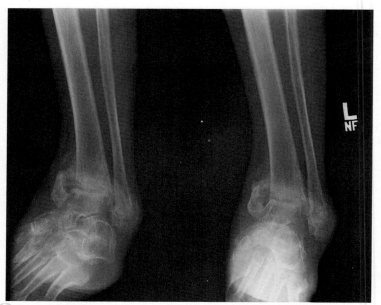

Figure **8-18.** ■ This image demonstrates multiple malalignments in the ankle of a patient with a Charcot's joint.

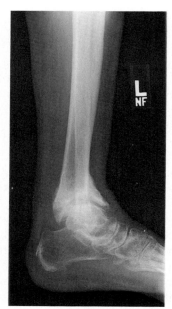

Figure **8-19.** ■ Charcot's joint. (1) Severe degenerative changes in the ankle joint. (2) Marked demineralization of the tarsals, to the point the trabecular patterns in the calcaneus are barely visible. (3) Inconsistent bone density in the tarsals.

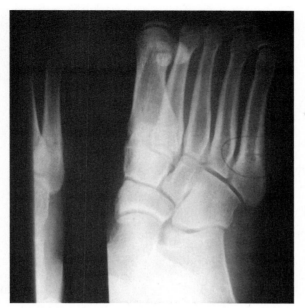

Figure 8-20 ■ AP of foot demonstrating Jones fracture of the fifth metatarsal.

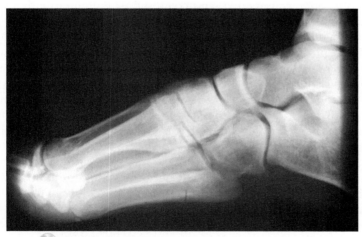

Figure 8-21. ■ Lateral of foot with Jones fracture.

progress to a nonunion or delayed union. Figures 8-20 and 8-21 demonstrate a Jones fracture, and Figure 8-22 shows a dancer's styloid avulsion fracture.

Avascular necrosis (AVN) in the foot and ankle can occur from trauma and or diseases. Fracture(s) to the talus may damage the blood supply to the talus and result in AVN.[8]

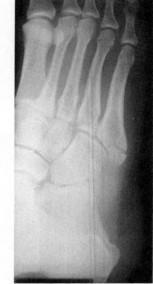

Figure **8-22.** ■ Medial oblique of foot demonstrating styloid fracture-avulsion fracture at insertion of peroneus brevis, also known as a "dancer's fracture."

Freiberg's infarction is AVN of the proximal second metatarsal. It occurs in females 3 or 4 to 1 over males, has a 13- to 18-year old age range, and is thought to be associated with overuse. On an AP x-ray, the head of the second metatarsal is sclerotic, often fragmented, and collapsed or flattening with a widening and thickening of the shaft.[9]

Early x-ray signs include flattening of the metatarsal head, progressing to fragmentation of the head, and a chronically painful joint (Figures 8-23 and 8-24).

Sever's disease is a calcaneal apophysitis, or painful inflammation, of the growth plate in preadolescents 8 to 12 years old. Plain films may demonstrate an increased distance in the width of the growth plate compared with the non-painful heel or may be unrevealing. The films will rule out other more worrisome diagnoses (Figure 8-25).

Stress Fractures

The causes of overuse are covered in depth in Chapter 6, but the foot sustains the highest number of stress fractures, most frequently in the metatarsals. The repetitive pounding sustained in running and jumping sports is seen in cross-country, track, soccer, basketball, and other sports. Refer to Figure 8-8, which demonstrates a healing callus or periosteal reaction on a third metatarsal stress fracture/reaction. See also Figures 8-26 to 8-30. The stress fracture or overuse injury in the fifth metatarsal is called a Jones fracture and is not to be confused with a styloid, or dancer's, fracture. Other examples of metatarsal fractures are shown in Figures 8-31 to 8-33.

The bones of the ankle and foot can be fractured by trauma, repetitive or acute, or diseases and/or pathologic weakening. Some examples are shown in Figures 8-34 to 8-49.

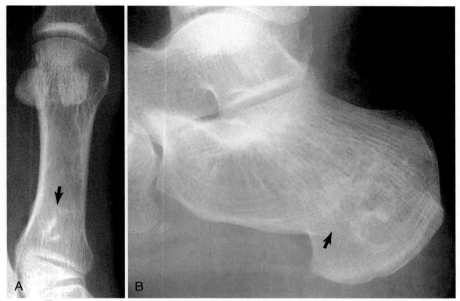

■ *Figure* **8-23.** ■ Osteonecrosis of diametaphyseal and irregular bones (the first metatarsal). *(From Christman RA:* Foot and ankle radiology, *London, 2003, Churchill Livingstone.)*

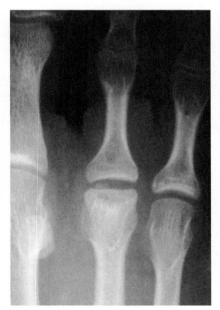

■ *Figure* **8-24.** ■ Demonstrates Freiberg's disease of proximal second metatarsal. *(From Green NE:* Skeletal Trauma in Children, *3e, Philadelphia, 2003, Saunders.)*

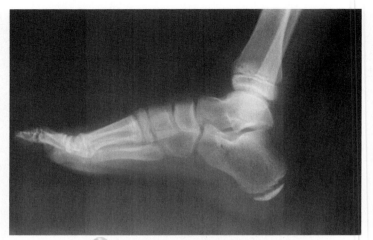

Figure 8-25. ■ Sever's disease.

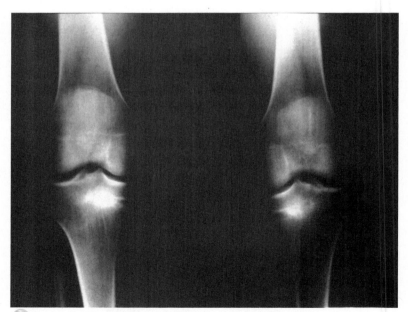

Figure 8-26. ■ Bilateral medial proximal stress reactions in a female runner.

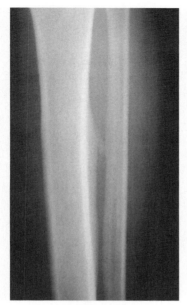

Figure 8-27. ■ Posterior midtibial healing callus in college female track athlete.

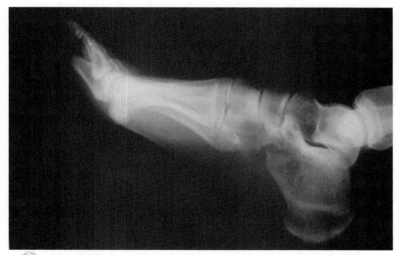

Figure 8-28. ■ Distal tibia stress reaction secondary to overuse.

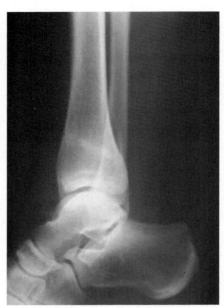

Figure **8-29.** ■ Stress reaction in the distal tibia. Note that the increased density in the distal tibia runs perpendicular to the trabeculae.

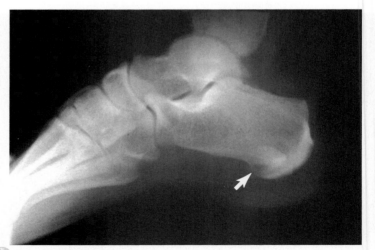

Figure **8-30.** ■ Stress reaction to distal tibia in runner. "Heel Spur" at attachment of the planar fascia.

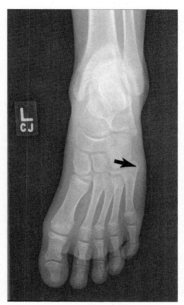

Figure 8-31. ■ AP of the foot in a child with a subtle fracture of the proximal styloid of the fifth metatarsal.

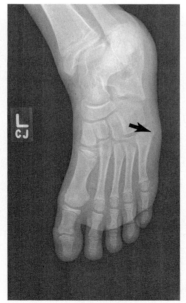

Figure 8-32. ■ Oblique view of a fifth metatarsal fracture. Avulsion fracture off the proximal styloid of the fifth metatarsal in a child. Very similar to a dancer's fracture/fracture of the styloid of the fifth metatarsal.

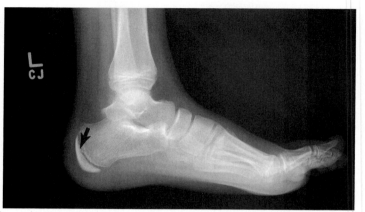

Figure 8-33. ■ Lateral view of a fifth metatarsal fracture. Sever's Disease: apophysitis of the distal calcaneal growth plate in an immature youth league football player.

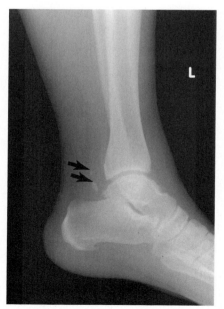

Figure 8-34. ■ Lateral view of calcification of posterior capsule of the ankle joint.

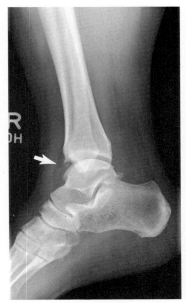

Figure 8-35. ■ Avulsion of medial malleolus, lateral view.

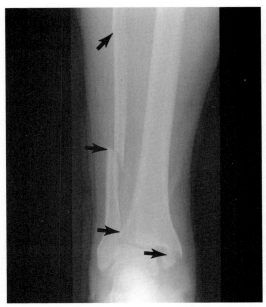

Figure 8-36. ■ Postreduction film of a dislocation of the ankle, prior to surgical stabilization. Note (1) the fracture of the fibula in two locations (2) the spread of the mortise (3) the fracture of the medial malleolus.

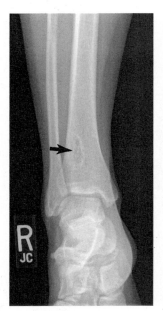

Figure 8-37. ■ Fibrous osseous lesion (in distal tibia), AP view.

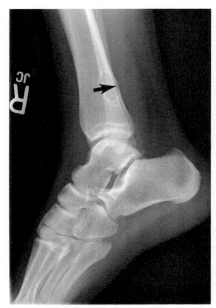

Figure 8-38. ■ Lateral view of a fiberous osseous lesion of the distal tibia. Note the posterior margin of the tibia is distorted and the bone is weakened in this region.

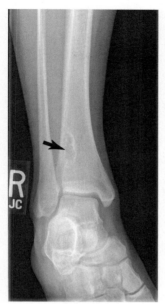

Figure 8-39. ■ Mortise view of a fiberous osseous lesion of the distal tibia. Note the margins of the lesion have an increased density compared to the surrounding bone.

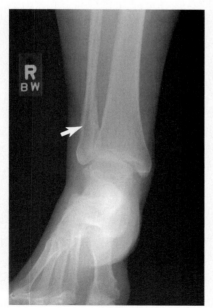

Figure 8-40. ■ Fibula fracture, AP view (demonstrating subtle compaction fracture of distal fibula).

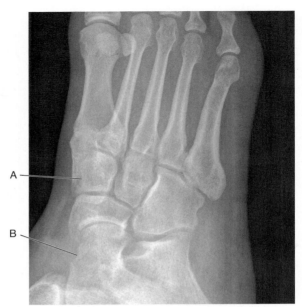

Figure 8-41. ■ **A,** Focal osteolysis of proximal navicular. **B,** distal talus.

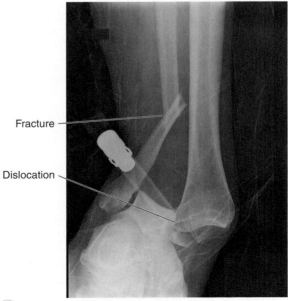

Figure 8-42. ■ Fracture dislocation, AP view of the right ankle.

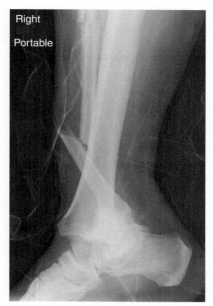

F*igure* 8-43. ■ Fracture dislocation, lateral view of the right ankle.

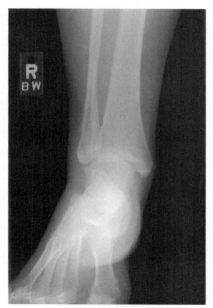

F*igure* 8-44. ■ AP view of a dislocated tibia but the lateral view is necessary to assess the extent of the dislocation.

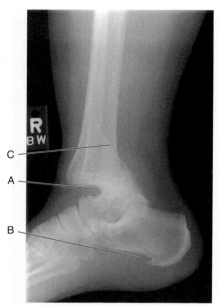

C

A

B

Figure 8-45. ■ Lateral view, **A,** posterior dislocation of foot on ankle. **B,** Note the heel spur on the calcaneus and **C,** fracture of the distal fibula.

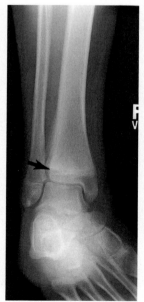

Figure 8-46. ■ Salter Harris fracture of distal tibia through the growth plate.

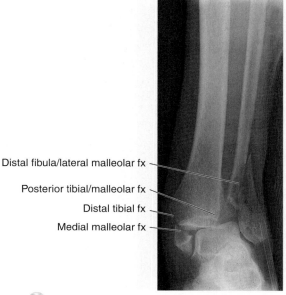

Distal fibula/lateral malleolar fx

Posterior tibial/malleolar fx

Distal tibial fx

Medial malleolar fx

Figure 8-47. ▪ AP view of 66-year-old female with a tri-malleolar fracture. Note distal fibula/lateral malleolar fracture, posterior tibial/malleolar fracture, distal tibial fracture and medial melleolar fracture.

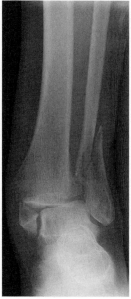

Figure 8-48. ▪ Trimalleolar fracture, AP view, 66-year-old female, mortise view.

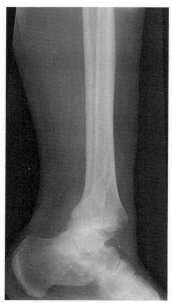

Figure 8-49. ■ Trimalleolar fracture, lateral view, 66-year-old female. Note the posterior subluxation of the talus.

Cartilage

Severe sprains, subluxations, dislocations, or direct trauma can chip off small (2 to 4 mm) sections of hyaline cartilage on the anterolateral or posteromedial surface of the talus. If not carefully evaluated, these osteochondral lesions are easily missed and may be a source of chronic pain in the ankle after severe sprain or trauma (Figures 8-50 and 8-51).

Soft Tissue

Major injuries in the foot may be fractures or dislocations because of the severity of the forces required to cause these injuries, but the trauma may also cause dislocations without osseous damage. These are relatively uncommon, but do occur. An example may be the inversion injury that compromises the lateral ligamentous complex leading to a chronically unstable ankle that will be symptomatically unstable under stress and in athletics, but be serviceable in normal gait on level surfaces.

To facilitate anatomic understanding, the foot is divided into the hindfoot, consisting of the talus and calcaneus; the midfoot, consisting of the navicular, cuboid, and the three cuneiform bones; and the forefoot, consisting of the metatarsals and the phalanges. Dislocations of the foot can occur in the midtarsal (Chopart's), tarsal-metatarsal (Lisfranc's), subtalar, or interphalangeal joint(s). The Lisfranc's joint sustains more dislocations than the other joints and accounts for approximately 1 in 50,000 of the orthopedic trauma cases annually, and the overwhelming majority of foot dislocations occur in males—6 times as often as females (Figure 8-52).

AP view   Mortise view

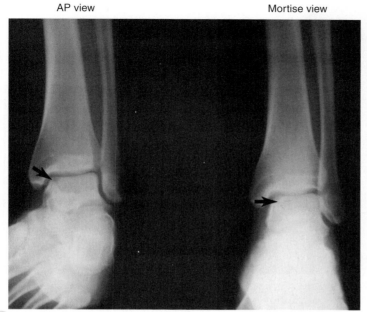

Figure 8-50. ■ A/P and mortise views showing OCDs on talar articular surface.

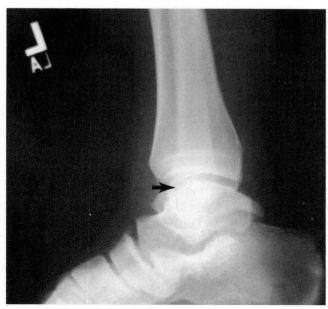

Figure 8-51. ■ Lateral view demonstrating a subtle osteochondral lesion in the talus. Note the subtle change in the density of the talus at the articular surface.

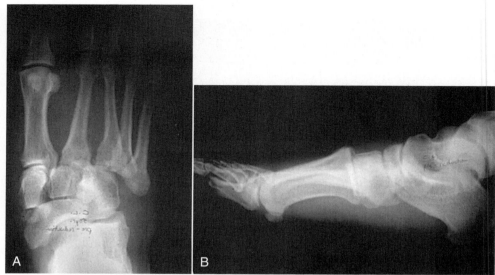

Figure 8-52. ■ Figure **A** is an AP of the Foot and Figure **B** is a lateral view. Note the disruption of alignment in both views at the tarsal-metatarsal line. In the AP view, the forefoot is shifted laterally, and in the lateral view, the forefoot is shifted dorsally. This is a Lisfranc dislocation. *(From Canale ST, Beaty JH:* Campbell's Operative Orthopedics, *11e, St. Louis, Mosby 2007)*

Whereas the ankle ligamentous complex is the tissue most often damaged in athletic endeavors, more than 95% of ankle sprains deal with the lateral ligaments. Soft tissue evaluation of the three standard views of the ankle is limited to any soft tissue swelling visible in the periarticular space. Often imaging or stress testing of the lateral ligament complex will reveal unacceptable laxity. The three standard views are supplemented with a stress view using a mechanical stress device that allows a film to be taken in neutral, then the joint is stressed in varus and the film is retaken. Measurements can then be made along the plafond and the talar surface on the uninvolved and the unstressed ankle and then remeasured after the involved ankle is stressed to allow comparison and a percent increase in motion (Figures 8-53 and 8-54).

Syndesmosis injuries may be a result of fibular fractures, fibular and medial malleolar fractures, or ligament damage from severe sprains. Damage to these structures results in the "high ankle sprain" much spoken about in the National Football League. Mechanisms of injury are dorsiflexion of the foot moving the talus into a "closed pack" position and accompanying forced external rotation of the foot (Figures 8-55 to 8-57).

The patient with a spread mortise from a severe sprain or a fracture will have difficulty bearing weight on the involved ankle and may show increased syndesmotic distance on plain films or stress views (Figures 8-58 to 8-60). Since the foot is not aligned in a true AP direction when the ankle dorsiflexes and plantar flexes, there is a rotational component to the movement. The method of stabilizing a spread mortise joint is with a transsyndesmotic screw

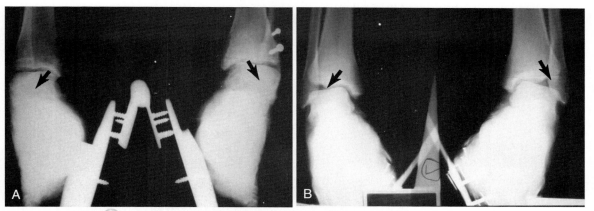

Figure 8-53. ■ Early version of the Telos Device to apply stress to the ankle joint to assess the stability of the joint. **A.** Note ORIF screws on left ankle. **B.** Note the measurable difference in the space between the joints.

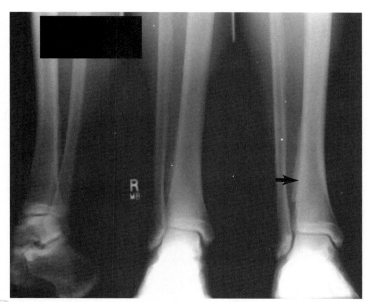

Figure 8-54. ■ Lateral, A/P, and mortise views of the ankle. Note only the mortise view demonstrates clearly the calcification of the interosseous ligament.

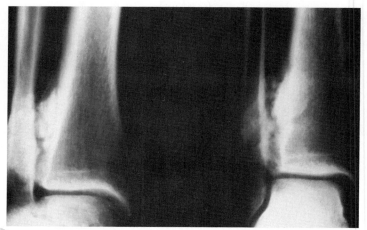

Figure 8-55. ■ A/P and mortise views of the ankle joint demonstrating calcification of the interosseous ligament.

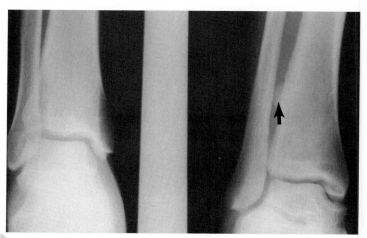

Figure 8-56. ■ A/P and mortise views of the ankle. Note the obvious calcification of the interosseous ligament visible on the mortise view but not so obvious on the A/P view.

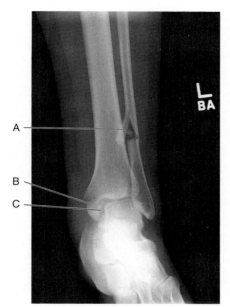

Figure 8-57. ■ AP view of a fibular fracture, medial malleolar fracture and spread of medial malleolar component of the mortise.

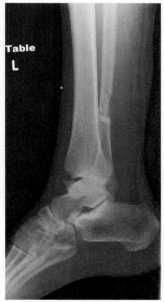

Figure 8-58. ■ Lateral view of the same fracture as 8-57.

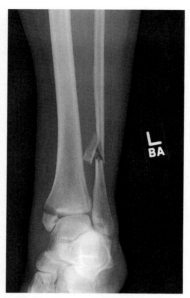

Figure 8-59. ■ Mortise view of the same fracture as 8-57 and 8-58. Take note of the clear spread of the mortise distance between the lateral distal tibia and the medial distal fibula. This joint will need ORIF to restore the integrity to the mortise joint.

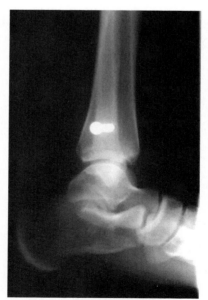

Figure 8-60. ■ Lateral view of a spread mortise that has been surgically reduced with a transsyndesmotic screw. Lateral view does not reveal that the screw was threaded the wrong direction and the rotation of the ankle joint caused it to back out of the bones.

Mortise   AP

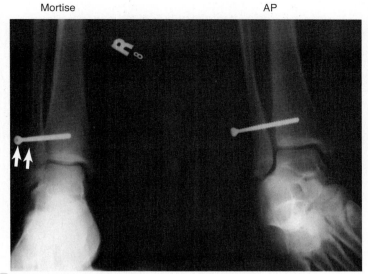

🔘 **Figure 8-61.** ■ A/P and mortise views of transsyndesmotic screw that has 'backed out' after 6 weeks. Normal position is through the 2 cortex bones of the fibula and tibia (4 total).

placed through all four cortices while the ankle is held in full dorsiflexion. The rotational component of movement mandates that there be screws that turn clockwise and counterclockwise. If a screw is placed that rotates in the opposite direction as the rotational component of that ankle, the screw will eventually back out (Figure 8-61).

Soft tissue swelling visible on any or all three standard ankle x-rays is an indication of significant soft tissue injury or an occult fracture and may require CT, MRI, or stress testing if the clinical exam warrants.

CASE STUDIES

CASE STUDY A

History: A 22-year-old wide receiver for a major college football team arrives in your clinic referred by his mother for difficulty "cutting when he plays football." "His ankle gives out." You evaluate him and have some questions about the stability of his ankle, so you request that his physician get some plain films taken. The films are viewed in the following sequence: Figure 8-62, 8-63, and 8-64.

What is your diagnosis? What are your recommendations?

Answer: He has marked instability on the lateral ligaments of the ankle, and he is referred to an orthopedic surgeon who rebuilds his lateral ankle and refers him back to you for postoperative rehabilitation.

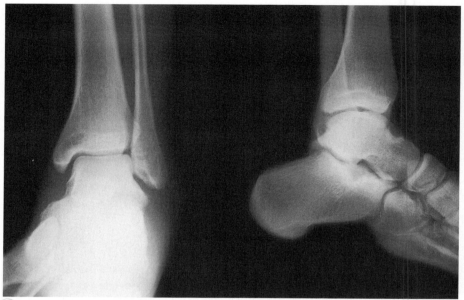

Figure 8-62. ■ AP and lateral views of a division I football player, a wide receiver, with inability to cut in one direction after a severe ankle sprain. His strength was excellent.

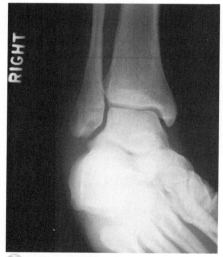

Figure 8-63. ■ Mortise view of patient in 8-62 is unremarkable.

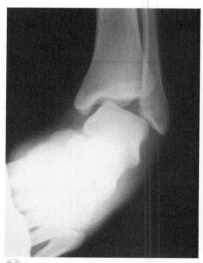

Figure 8-64. ■ Stress tested view of the lateral ankle demonstrating clearly that his inability to cut off this ankle is a result of the complete compromise of his lateral ligamentous complex and static stability.

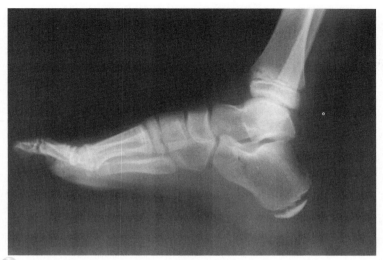

Figure 8-65. ■ Lateral view of the ankle in a 10 year old boy football player with difficulty bearing weight on the foot, particularly the heel. Pain with active resisted plantar flexion x-ray confirms acute apophysitis or also referred to as Sever's disease.

CASE STUDY B

History: A 10-year-old male playing "Pop Warner" football begins to limp on his right foot at practice, and his parents bring him into your clinic after having an x-ray taken at a quick clinic. The film is a lateral view (Figure 8-65). Upon arrival in your clinic, he is walking on the ball of his right foot with decreased stance on the right. He is hesitant to dorsiflex his right ankle fully, and motor function and sensation are intact. He is extremely tender to palpation on the right distal ankle.

What is your diagnosis? What are your recommendations?

Answer: This boy has Sever's disease, an apophysitis of the growth plate in the calcaneus from overuse. The treatment is rest, heel cup, weight bearing to tolerance, cross-training with water therapy, upper body exercises, taping may help, tincture of time, and gradual resumption of activities.

CASE STUDY C

History: A 24-year-old skydiver lands extremely hard on his heel from a jump and experiences an immediate onset of severe pain and swelling in his ankle and inability to bear weight. The lateral film is unrevealing, but the AP demonstrates the pathologic condition, as does the CT (Figure 8-66).

What is your diagnosis? What are your recommendations?

Answer: Fracture of the talus. Two concerns are AVN and displacement of the fracture resulting in severe arthritis of the ankle in the future. This patient needs management by an orthopedic surgeon on an emergency basis. Refer to surgeon of choice or an emergency room.

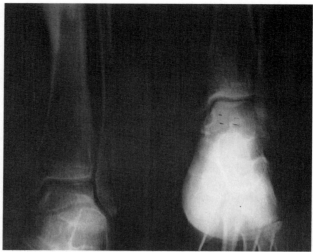

***Figure* 8-66.** ■ AP of the foot in a patient who had a parachute failure on his jump resulting in a high impact fall onto his foot and ankle. Bone exam demonstrates a fracture of the talus bone and severe soft tissue swelling.

REFERENCES

1. O'Keeffe D et al: ABC of emergency radiology: "the ankle," *BMJ* 308:331, 1994.
2. Resnick D, Niwayama G: *Diagnosis of bone and joint disorders,* ed 2, Philadelphia, 1988, WB Saunders.
3. Bozzelle JR: e-Medicine, retrieved at www.emedicine.com/orthoped/topic279.htm. Updated Feb 15, 2008.
4. Netter FH: *The Ciba collection of medical illustrations, musculoskeletal system,* Vol 8 part 1. Icon Learning systems, Yardly PA 1994
5. Evans MJ, Schucany WG: Radiological evaluation of a high ankle sprain, Vol 19(4) Oct 2006 pp 402-405 *Baylor University Medical Center Proc.*
6. Christman RA: *Foot and ankle radiology,* St Louis, 2003, Elsevier.
7. Avascular necrosis and related disorders of the foot and ankle, http://www.nwhealth. edu/conted/distlear/AVN/avnfoot.html Northwest University, 2001. Last viewed June 16, 2008.
8. McStay CM: Dislocations of the foot, *eMedicine* p 2, April 2006. http://www.emedicine. com/EMERG/topic141.htm Last accessed June 16, 2008.
9. Lin CF, Gross MT, Weinhold P: Ankle syndesmosis injuries: anatomy, biomechanics, mechanism of injury and clinical guidelines for diagnosis and intervention. *JOSPT* (36):6, 372-384, 2006.

9 The Shoulder

INTRODUCTION

Remarks

Although it is not within the scope of this book to provide a complete anatomic review of each segment covered, the shoulder is so unique that a few brief comments are appropriate to review the critical components and considerations of this joint. This joint is the most mobile joint in the body and as such is the most susceptible to problems of instability. The causes of these instabilities can be trauma, congenital defect, or disease related. The shoulder is almost entirely dependent upon the support of the surrounding soft tissue structures, specifically the contractile tissue of the rotator cuff, the joint capsule, and the glenoid labrum for its stability.

In comparison with the hip, which is a weight-bearing joint with an inherent structural stability, the shoulder literally hangs on the rotator cuff, levered against the glenoid fossa with some increased surface area provided by the fibrocartilaginous labrum (the meniscus of the shoulder) and supported by the muscles connecting to the rotator cuff. Witness the devastating effect on the integrity of this joint that a motor cortex cerebral vascular accident has when it leaves the cuff paralyzed or the effect of a peripheral nerve injury that damages one or all of the upper brachial plexus nerves that supply the muscles of this joint.

It is important while viewing the x-ray film depictions of this joint that the interpreter projects onto the film the things that can be seen only in his or her mind, the soft tissue structures, which comprise the support systems for this joint. The healthy shoulder capsule attaches to the humeral head at the anatomical neck and to the lateral portion of the neck of the glenoid and provides stability and restraint to the glenohumeral joint while allowing a full range of motion (ROM). There is a thickening in the capsule, the long head of the biceps that passes through the capsule, but is encased in the synovium. It is therefore intracapsular but extrasynovial. The long head of the triceps attaches to the inferior surface of the glenoid and along with the long head of the biceps creates an additional muscular or contractile tissue support system for the joint.

The shoulder joint consists of: (1) the proximal humeral bone and the glenoid of the scapula that form the glenohumeral joint, (2) the distal clavicle and the acromion that form the acromioclavicular (AC) joint, and (3) the medial components of the scapula and the proximal, lateral rib cage that form the scapulothoracic joint.

Scapulothoracic rhythm is the description given to the precise neuromuscular control in the shoulder musculature that creates the movement that allows the shallow glenoid to rotate clockwise on the left side and counterclockwise on the right side along and around the rib cage to maintain the glenoid in a position to articulate with and support the proximal humerus as it is abducted and flexed through its 180 degree arc. The proximal humerus and the scapula are both cancellous bone that when healthy are seen with normal bony margins and consistent density throughout the trabecular patterns.

OBJECTIVES ■■■■■■■

1. Recall the seven standard views of the shoulder and AC joint and their purposes.
2. Identify the normal and abnormal alignment in the seven standard views of the shoulder and AC joint.
3. Identify the normal and abnormal densities of the shoulder.
4. Identify the normal and abnormal cartilage.
5. Identify the normal and abnormal presentation of soft tissue.
6. Identify film abnormalities, given a history and x-ray film.
7. Use that information to adjust a physical therapy (PT) treatment program, given x-ray film abnormalities.

STANDARD VIEWS

Glenohumeral Joint

Standard views of the glenohumeral joint are anteroposterior (AP) projections in the following positions.

Anteroinferior Lateral (Resnick[1]) or AP in External Rotation (McKinnis[2]) (Figure 9-1)

Abduction Internal Rotation (Figure 9-2)

Lateral or Transscapular View (Figures 9-3 and 9-4)

The lateral or transscapular view is used to assess the integrity of the glenohumeral joint. It is taken so that the beam traverses the scapula and glenohumeral joint, depicting a series of concentric shapes from the most medial to the most lateral, with the innermost shape consisting of the glenoid and

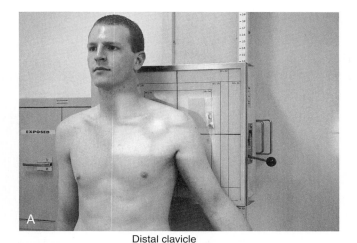

Distal clavicle

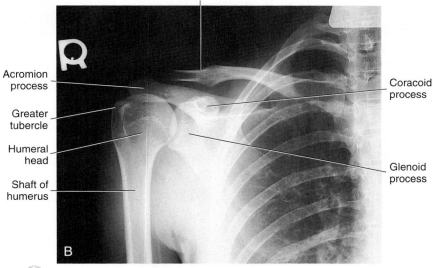

Acromion
process

Greater
tubercle

Humeral
head

Shaft of
humerus

Coracoid
process

Glenoid
process

Figure 9-1. ■ The position for taking an AP view of the shoulder with
the arm in an externally rotated position. *(From Long BW, Frank ED, Erlich
RA:* Radiography essentials for limited practice, *ed 2, 2006, Saunders.)*

concentrically around it the margins of the humeral head and both centered on
the axis created by the branching of the scapula into the inferior surface, anteriorly the coracoid, and posteroproximally the spine of the scapula terminating
in the acromion.

West Point View (Figures 9-5 and 9-6)

This west point view is used to visualize the glenoid rim and the relationship
of the proximal humerus to the glenoid. It is taken with the patient prone and
the arm at the 90-90 position, with the beam angled from 25 degrees cephalad
and 25 degrees lateral to medial. It is particularly useful when there is a suspicion

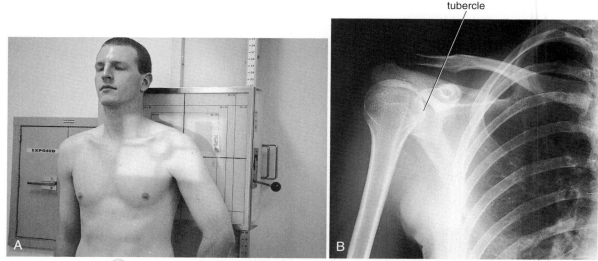

Lesser
tubercle

Figure 9-2. ■ The position for taking an AP view of the shoulder with the arm internally rotated to allow visualization of the proximal humerus at approximately a 90-degree different angle than the standard AP view with external rotation. *(From Long BW, Frank ED, Erlich RA:* Radiography essentials for limited practice, *ed 2, 2006, Saunders.)*

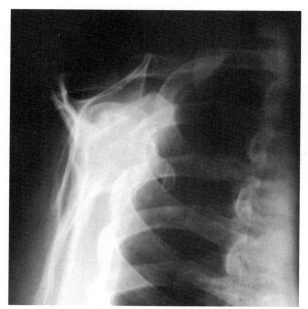

Figure 9-3. ■ **The effect of a transscapular view of the glenohu-meral joint.** Note the "Y" shape of the scapula formed by the scapular spine, the acromion, and the inferior blade of the scapula and the round humeral head covering the intersection of the "Y."

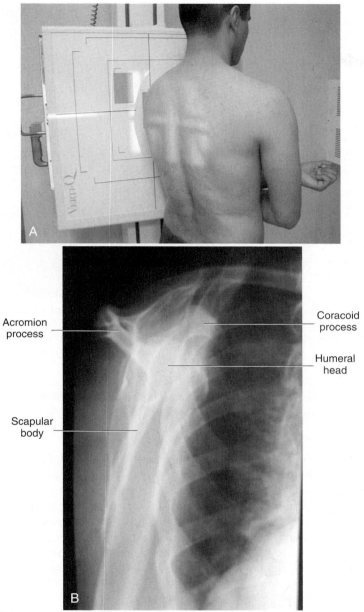

Acromion
process

Scapular
body

Coracoid
process

Humeral
head

Figure 9-4. ■ Patient position necessary to take a transscapular view. *(From Long BW, Frank ED, Erlich RA:* Radiography essentials for limited practice, *ed 2, 2006, Saunders.)*

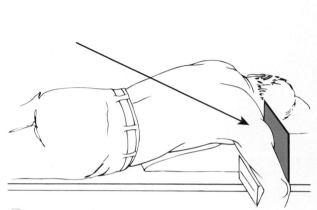

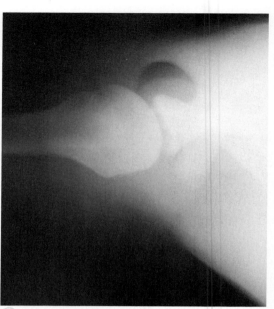

Figure **9-5.** ■ Patient position necessary to take a West Point view of the shoulder. *(From Browner B, Jupiter J, Trafton P:* Skeletal trauma: basic science, management, and reconstruction, *ed 3, 2003, Saunders.)*

Figure **9-6.** ■ **The result of a West Point view of the glenohumeral joint.** Note the acromion superior to the glenoid and the coracoid process, which is inferior to the glenoid in this view.

of a previous history of instability and will sometimes demonstrate a "Bankart lesion" that may not be visible on the standard AP projection.

AC Joint

The AC joint consists of the articulation created by the distal clavicle and the distal acromion. Its integrity hinges upon the coracoclavicular ligaments, the conoid and the trapezoid, which hold the clavicle in proximity to the conoid coracoacromial ligament of the scapula. Instability or tearing of these ligaments will allow the distal section of the clavicle to shift cephalad as seen in AC separations of this joint. The cause of this injury is a fall onto the shoulder that depresses the acromion to the level that the clavicle is held immobile. Continued acromion caudal movement tears the conoid, trapezoid and coracoacromial ligaments.

AP View (Figure 9-7)

The standard view of the AC joint is taken with the patient seated, and the beam travels in an AP direction, but angled 15 degrees in a cephalad direction.[1]

Weighted View (Figure 9-8)

Special views of the AC joint are two views taken in an AP projection: (1) with weights (WW) hung from the patient's wrists to depress the AC joint without causing the muscle stabilization that holding the weights in

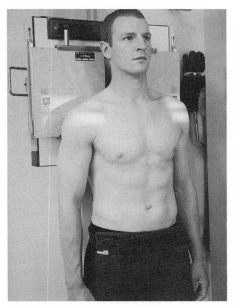

Figure 9-7. ■ Patient position necessary to take an AP view of the AC joint. *(From Long BW, Frank ED, Erlich RA:* Radiography essentials for limited practice, *ed 2, 2006, Saunders.)*

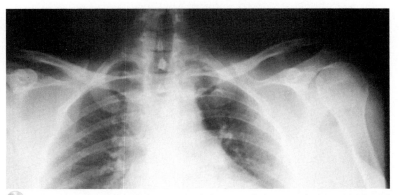

Figure 9-8. ■ Note the increased distance between the coracoid and clavicle on one side versus the other. Note the changes in the density of lung tissue. Note the deviation of the distal trachea, which is not pathologic.

their hands might cause and (2) without weights (WOW). An x-ray film that includes both the affected and unaffected shoulders allows measurement and comparison of the distance between the inferior margin of the clavicles and the respective cephalad edges of the coracoid processes on each side.

EVALUATION OF THE SHOULDER USING ABCS

Glenohumeral Joint

AP View

Alignment

Normal alignment (Figure 9-9). The alignment in the shoulder is assessed by the evaluation of the relationship of the humeral head to the glenoid. Is there slight overlap of the medial humeral head with the posterior glenoid? Are there more than 7 to 8 mm between the superior portion of the humeral head and the inferior surface of the acromion? Is the distal clavicle aligned with the acromion?

Abnormal alignment. Rotator Cuff tear (Figure 9-10): Less than 7 to 8 mm may indicate a subluxation of the humeral head up through the rotator cuff proximally toward the acromion. This occurs in a large tear.

Glenohumeral dislocation or subluxation (Figure 9-11): Glenohumeral instabilities can be divided into loose connective and/or capsular tissue, subluxations, and dislocations. Subluxations and dislocations are in the antero inferior direction more than 97% of the time, with occasional posterosuperior and multidirectional dislocations.[3] In an anteroinferior dislocation, the humeral head is inferior relative to its normal alignment with the glenoid, and in a posterior

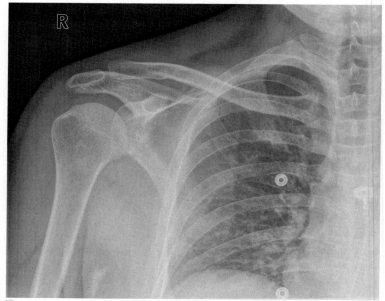

Figure **9-9.** ■ **AP view of a normal shoulder.** Note the alignment of the humeral head with the glenoid fossa and the relationship of the distal clavicle with the acromion. The humeral head has a well-demarcated space below the acromion for the rotator cuff.

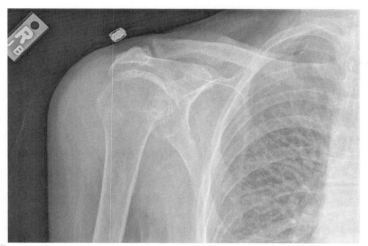

Figure 9-10. ■ Note the lack of subacromial space, indicating a rotator cuff tear. Also note the irregular shape of the humeral head from degenerative changes.

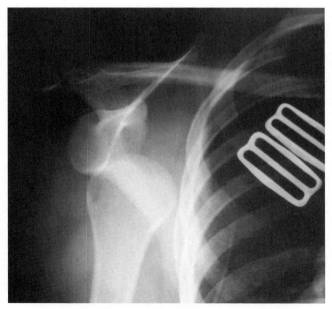

Figure 9-11. ■ Note that the humeral head is not aligned with the glenoid fossa, but is inferior to it and adjacent to the ribs. This patient has an inferiorly dislocated shoulder.

dislocation, the humeral head can usually be visualized as overlapping the proximal portion of the glenoid. Figure 9-12 demonstrates the same shoulder as Figure 9-11 after reduction of the dislocation.

Subluxation and loose collagen or connective tissue instabilities can be diagnosed with a clinical examination, including the apprehension sign, sulcus sign, drawer sign, and Feagin test. (Figure 9-13).

Bone

Normal bone. Are there consistent trabecular and cancellous patterns in the humeral head and the glenoid? Evaluate the bones for areas of increased or decreased density and lines of decreased density that may indicate occult, nondisplaced fractures. Cystic changes indicate severe degenerative changes in the bone. Age is not a prerequisite for these. Occasionally an athlete with a history of chronic instability of the glenohumeral joint will develop these changes, usually accompanied by osteophytosis. Does the metaphysis merge seamlessly with the epiphysis, and are the edges of the shaft of the humeral cortical bone visibly uninterrupted?

Abnormal bone. A Hill-Sachs lesion or deformity can occur in the superolateral or the posterolateral aspect of the humeral head when the dislocated humeral head is impacted against the anteroinferior edge of the glenoid in an anteroinferior dislocation (Figure 9-14).[1,4] This impaction can cause a divot or lesion shaped like a shallow wedge or "hatchet defect" in the humeral head.[4] These can be more challenging to reduce because of the bony impaction and the

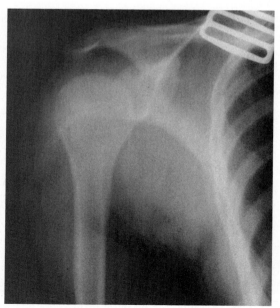

Figure **9-12.** ■ **Same patient shown in Figure 9-11.** Note that the humerus is now congruent with the glenoid fossa.

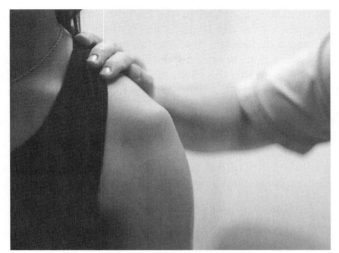

Figure 9-13. ■ If an individual has a lax capsule and recurrent dislocations of the shoulder, it may be possible to demonstrate this with a sulcus test. If the patient relaxes while traction is exerted in an inferior direction, it may be possible to see a depression or sulcus at the glenohumeral joint. *(DeLee J, Drez D, Miller M:* DeLee and Drez's orthopedic sports medicine, *ed 2, 2003, Saunders.)*

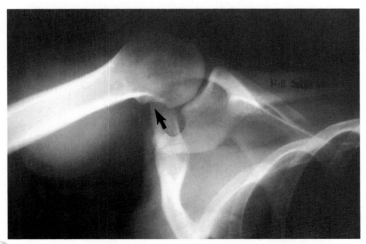

Figure 9-14. ■ The *black arrow* points to a defect in the humeral head where it impacted on the glenoid rim during a shoulder dislocation. This defect is called a Hill-Sachs lesion.

accompanying muscle spasm that holds the humeral head against the rim of the glenoid (Figures 9-15 and 9-16, see also Figure 9-11).

Note that during a dislocation, the insertion of the supraspinatus can remain attached and avulse a bony fragment from its insertion on the greater tuberosity of the humerus. That this fragment can remain attached by the periosteum demonstrates the strength of the periosteum. Once the shoulder is reduced, the fragment normally is reduced (Figures 9-17 to 9-19).

Fractures can be classified or described by: site and extent, type of fracture, alignment of fragments, direction of fracture line, consequence(s) of the fracture on the remaining bone (impacted, depressed, compressed), associated pathologic conditions (fracture dislocation), and the consequences to the joints involved based on the patient's age (Salter-Harris, hip fractures, and fracture dislocations in the elderly).[3]

Shaft of Humerus (Figures 9-20 to 9-22): Bone when subjected to a stress over a short unit of time will tolerate much higher stress for that short period than the same bone subjected to lower stress over a longer unit of time. If the stress exceeds the stress tolerance for that shorter unit of time, the bone shatters into comminuted fragments.

Surgical Neck. The surgical neck of the humerus is the proximal metaphyseal region where the shaft of the humerus/diaphysis transitions to the head of the humerus. (Figure 9-23):

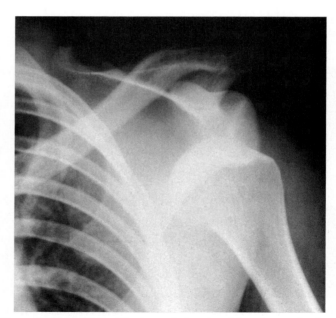

Figure **9-15.** ■ This AP view of the shoulder shows the humeral head to be inferior to the glenoid fossa, demonstrating a dislocated shoulder.

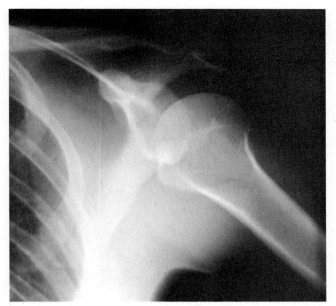

Figure 9-16. ■ **This AP view of the glenohumeral joint shows the humeral head inferior to the complete glenoid fossa.** The striking of the humeral head on the edge of the glenoid can cause a Hill-Sachs lesion.

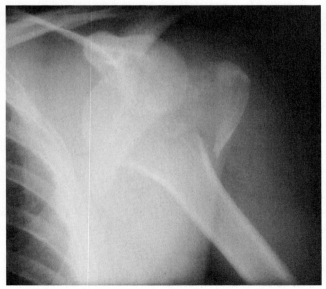

Figure 9-17. ■ This AP view of the shoulder shows a large fragment of the humeral head broken off with the remainder of the humeral head inferior to the glenoid fossa, showing a fracture dislocation.

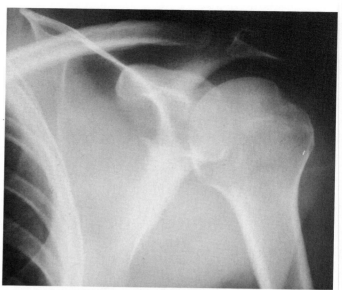

Figure 9-18. ■ **This film demonstrates the same shoulder shown in Figure 9-17 after reduction of the fracture and dislocation.** The periosteum of the humerus has pulled the fragments back into place after shoulder reduction to the point that on this AP view, the fracture is no longer evident.

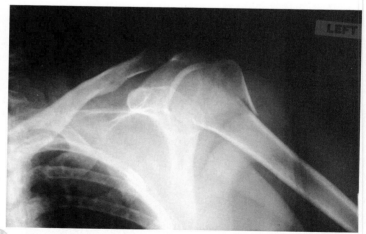

Figure 9-19. ■ **This shoulder view shows appropriate alignment of the humeral head with the glenoid fossa.** However, when tracing the margins of the humerus, there is a small discontinuity at the superior intersection of the humeral shaft with the humeral head. The individual has suffered an impacted fracture of the humeral head. The shaft of the humerus has been driven into the humeral head. This type of fracture when healed often results in very little or no disability if the articular surface of the humerus was not disrupted. Clinical relevance: no manual traction on this humeral shaft.

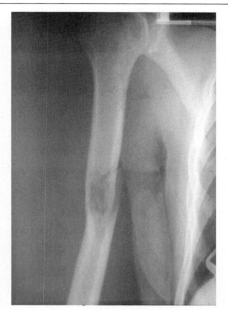

Figure 9-20. ■ Note the fracture of the midshaft of the humerus. Also note the decreased density of uneven margins in the bone at the level of the fracture, indicating a pathologic fracture.

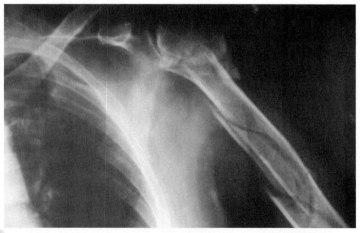

Figure 9-21. ■ Note the comminuted fracture of the diaphysis of the humerus that runs from the surgical neck along the shaft of the bone. Note that the fracture fragments are being maintained in some semblance of proximity to one another by the strong fibrous periosteum. This fracture also demonstrates the principle of the viscoelasticity of bone as per Dr. Frankel's studies.

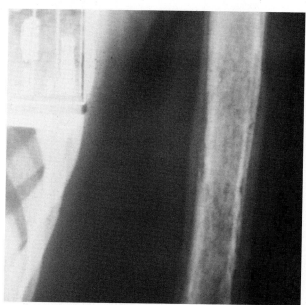

Figure 9-22. ■ **This film depicts sickle cell sludging in the vessels of the humerus during a "crisis."** Note the widespread necrotic areas in the humeral bone where the sludging stopped the vascular flow to the bony tissue. Take special note of how the periosteum is swollen and lifted from the cortical edges of the bone.

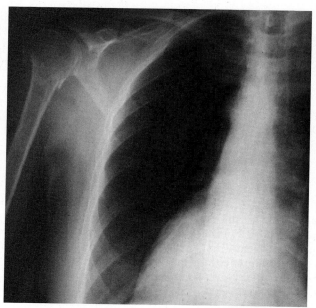

Figure 9-23. ■ **An impacted fracture of the surgical neck.** The patient is usually treated with a sling. Do not apply traction to the injury.

Scapula: The patient in Figures 9-24 to 9-26 sustained a fracture of the inferior glenoid and dislocation during a fall from a treadmill in the gymnasium. It represents a Bankart fracture. Figure 9-24 is from an early computed tomography (CT) scan.

Within a week after surgery, this patient was sent to PT with a referral that gave his diagnosis, frequency, and duration of treatment and orders to "not let his shoulder get stiff." Please devise a treatment plan for this injury and compare it with the treatment plan you would have devised for the impacted fracture (nonpathologic fracture) of the surgical neck of the humerus (Figures 9-27 and 9-28).

Clinical question: How would you treat the following patient in the clinic? The patient is 2 weeks post fracture and arrives in the clinic with a referral requesting "PT, evaluate and treat, 3 × week for 3 weeks." Is the humeral head a smooth, uninterrupted, hemispherical shape? Evaluate the AC joint for cystic and or degenerative changes and evidence of fracture or separation. Review the margins of the visible portions of the ribs and the scapula (Figures 9-29 to 9-31).

Cartilage

Normal cartilage. Cartilage in the shoulder refers to the articular cartilage on the humeral head and the articular surface of the glenoid and the fibrocartilage of the glenoid labrum.

Abnormal cartilage. The absence of articular cartilage in the glenohumeral joint is suggested by clinical signs and symptoms of pain and joint crepitation that accompany movement and by bone-on-bone ratcheting that may be felt

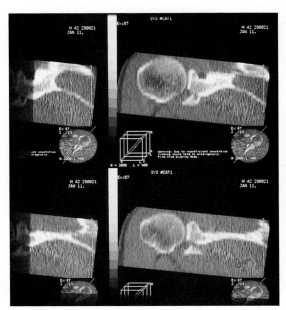

Figure 9-24. ■ **CT scan of the glenohumeral joint.** Note in all images that a portion of the glenoid has been fractured.

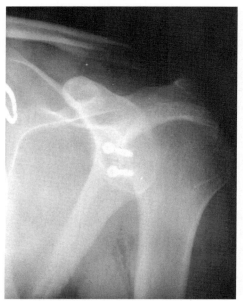

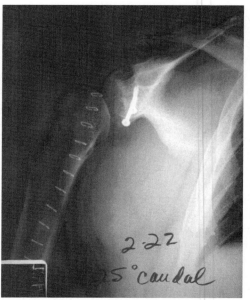

Figure **9-25.** ■ Open reduction internal fixation (ORIF) of an inferior scapular fragment.

Figure **9-26.** ■ Metallic staples used to close skin and the metallic screws used to secure the fragment back to the scapula.

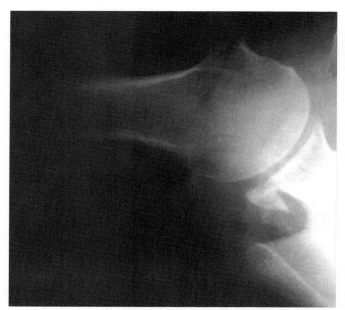

Figure **9-27.** ■ Plain film x-ray in an axillary or West Point View of a fracture of the glenoid, a Bankart fracture.

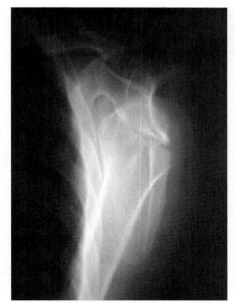

F*igure* 9-28. ■ Transscapular view demonstrating a scapular fracture.

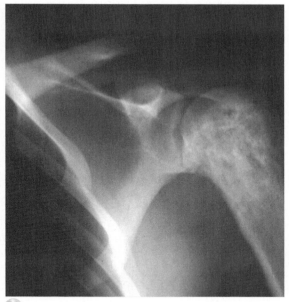

F*igure* 9-29. ■ **Plain x-ray film of Ewing's sarcoma in a 14-year-old male.** The patient had been sent to PT for "shoulder pain" and repeatedly sent back to the orthopedic resident for "increasing shoulder pain without relief from therapy." Note the "moth-eaten" looking lesions in the proximal humerus.

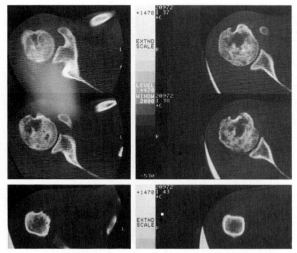

F*igure* 9-30. ■ **A CT scan of the same patient shown in Figure 9-29.** Note the irregular margins of the medullary canal and "chewed-up" appearance of the humeral head bone. No consistent bony trabecular patterns are present. The bone is full of lytic lesions.

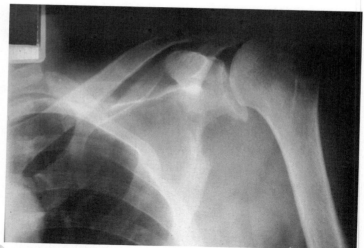

Figure 9-31. ■ Note the missing portion of the lateral scapula, inferior to the glenoid. This is a lytic tumor of the scapula.

and heard as the patient attempts to move his or her arm through its ROM. This is occasionally visible on the x-ray films as decreased space in the joint, osteophytosis and/or cystic formation in the humeral head or glenoid. A torn labrum can be expected to accompany a history of instability that includes a dislocation and will sometimes be visible on x-ray films as an osteophyte on the anteroinferior edge of the glenoid, a form of the Bankart lesion (Figure 9-32).

Soft Tissue

Normal soft tissue. Soft tissue is evaluated in the shoulder by carefully viewing the visible portions of the soft tissue that surround the shoulder and the

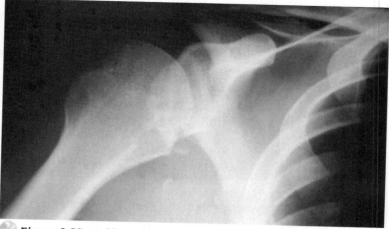

Figure 9-32. ■ Note the osteophyte inferior to the glenoid fossa. This is a Bankart lesion.

visible portion of the lung. Any change in the density of the lung or inconsistency visualized must be explained or followed up. Carefully assess the relationship between the top of the humeral head and the inferior portion of the acromion (Figure 9-33).

Abnormal soft tissue. Rotator cuff pathologic conditions: Rotator cuff pathologic conditions are an extremely common problem with people over 50 years old. Tears of the cuff do occur traumatically in younger athletes and as the result of trauma from severe falls—as occur in skiing and mountain biking, vehicular accidents, football, etc.—but not to the extent that they do in the older population. The older the patient, the higher the risk they have for rotator cuff pathology.

The muscular component of the rotator cuff that serves the glenohumeral joint is made up of the supraspinatus, infraspinatus, and teres minor, which insert on the superior and posterior portion of the greater tuberosity, and the subscapularis, which inserts on the lesser tuberosity of the humerus anteriorly. The insertional tendons of these muscles form the rotator cuff.

When in proper tone and undamaged, these muscles provide concentric, eccentric, and isometric control and contribute greatly to the stability and proper function of the glenohumeral joint. Electromyographic studies have proven that as the humeral head begins motion into abduction the muscles of the cuff, particularly the supraspinatus, pull the humeral head into firm contact with the glenoid and depress the humeral head, thereby preventing impingement of the superior cuff muscles and the head onto the inferior surface and edge of the acromion. Without this precise functional neuromuscular timing, the joint is traumatized repeatedly (Figure 9-34). Critical to the understanding of the

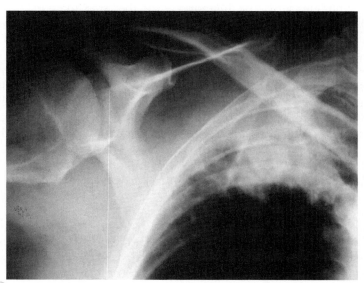

Figure **9-33.** ■ Examine the lung field in this view. The increased density in the upper portion of the lung is a tumor.

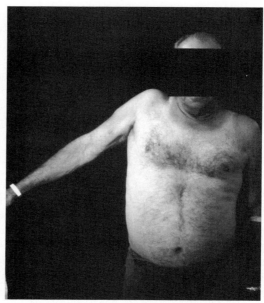

Figure 9-34. ■ The patient is unable to abduct his arm as a result of a torn rotator cuff. He was also incapable of active abduction.

pathologic conditions of the rotator cuff is the anatomic understanding that the superior border of the supraspinatus is contiguous with the inferior surface of the subacromial bursa.

Before the advent of diagnostic orthopedic ultrasonography and magnetic resonance imaging (MRI), the diagnostic test—the "sine qua non" if you will—for a tear in the rotator cuff was a contrast shoulder arthrogram (Figure 9-35). Dye was injected into the shoulder capsule, distributed with air, and the joint mobilized to ensure spread of the dye, and an x-ray was taken of the shoulder (Figure 9-36). The essential diagnostic element for a torn cuff was dye leaking into the subacromial bursa. If the dye leaked, the cuff had to be torn. If the dye did not leak, the cuff or at least enough of the cuff to prevent leakage was intact. A massive tear could allow the dye to leak all the way into the subdeltoid bursa. Successful rehabilitation of the cuff after repair depends upon the size of the tear, repair technique, length of time the cuff was torn before it was addressed surgically, and the condition of the muscular components of the cuff.

The state of the art imaging at this time is noninvasive ultrasonography or MRI for diagnosis of a torn rotator cuff. Of the two, the MRI is more expensive, but more accurate.

A notable decrease in the subacromial space, less than 7-8 mm may be diagnostic of a large tear of the rotator cuff. Folds or creases in the surrounding soft tissue can create lucencies that may appear as lines of decreased density in the bony tissue. These can be traced carefully to ensure that they exceed the margins of the bone(s) without interruption, indicating that they are not contained solely within the bone and are not an occult, nondisplaced fracture.

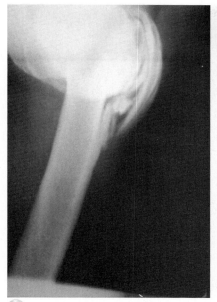

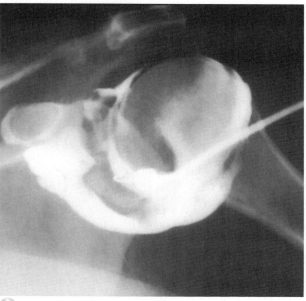

Figure 9-35. ■ A normal arthrogram with dye in the shoulder. Note the extent of the normal capsule.

Figure **9-36.** ■ A needle in the shoulder capsule to deliver dye.

Calcification of the supraspinatus tendon: Calcification of the supraspinatus tendon is speculated to be the result of chronic impingement, overuse, etc. Studies indicate that not all people with calcification of the supraspinatus tendon have painful shoulders, but those who do are at an increased risk of developing pain compared with the population that does not have this calcification of the tendon. It is critical to remember that on standard-routine films of the shoulder the subacromial space is not well visualized when the film is hanging on a view box. However, if the film is held up to a "hot light," the space becomes well illuminated, and the calcification of the tendon that may not have been visible becomes obvious (Figure 9-37).

Lateral or Transscapular View

The purpose of the lateral view is to determine the relationship of the humeral head to the glenoid. The alignment of the humeral head is the primary purpose of this view.

Alignment

Normal alignment. The coracoid process, the acromion process, and the blade of the scapula form a "Y" shape, or Mercedes-Benz type sign. The round head of the humerus should be superimposed in the middle of the Y (see Figure 9-3).

Abnormal alignment. When assessing a total shoulder arthroplasty (TSA), because the joint has been painful for so long before the surgery and the joint now has significantly reduced proprioception means that the patient may be unaware of the joint's instability or frank dislocation. In this situation, a lateral scapular, or transscapular, view may be extremely revealing (Figure 9-38).

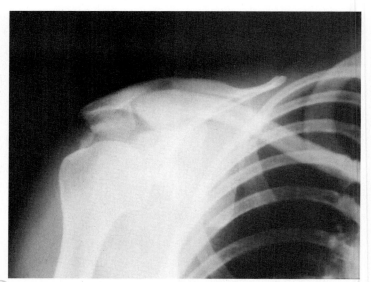

Figure **9-37.** ■ Note the calcification of the supraspinatus tendon in the subacromial space.

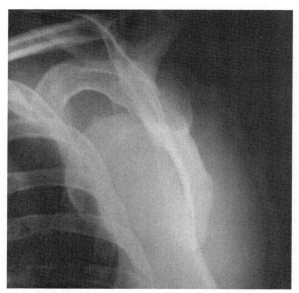

Figure **9-38.** ■ **The transscapular or lateral view of the scapula along the blade of the scapular spine.** The coracoid process arches to the left, and the acromion process arches to the right in this view. The humeral head should be centered on the intersection of the coracoid, the acromion, and the spinous processes. In this view, the humeral head is inferior and medial to its normal position, demonstrating a shoulder dislocation.

The AP view does not clearly demonstrate that this shoulder is dislocated, and the patient was not aware that it was dislocated and had been for some time (Figure 9-39). The clinical indication was that the patient could not progress beyond about 90 degrees of forward flexion in spite of intensive PT. The shoulder had been in this condition for more than 10 years. The patient's pain was minimal, and she made excellent initial progress in therapy until she plateaued at 90 degrees. Note on the transscapular view in Figure 9-40 that the humerus is anterior to the holes that anchor the invisible glenoid portion of the prosthesis to the glenoid just above and below the intersection of the "Y" created by the lateral projection of the scapula.

Posterior dislocations can be difficult to distinguish from the anteroinferior dislocations on the standard AP projections. The lateral, or transscapular, projection is invaluable if the clinical presentation does not make the position obvious. Clinically, rehabilitation of a shoulder with a history of acute shoulder dislocation may be designed differently to emphasize different muscles for an anterior verses a posterior dislocation.

Bone
Normal bone
Abnormal bone. Cartilage and soft tissue are not observable in this view.
West Point or Axillary View
At times the West Point view will demonstrate a bony Bankart lesion when a standard view is not conclusive (Figure 9-41).

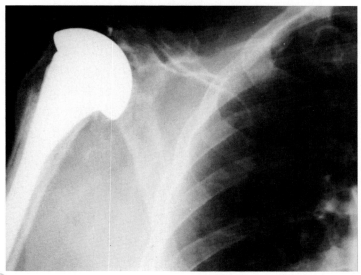

⬤ *Figure* **9-39.** ■ **An AP view of a shoulder following an arthroplasty.** The glenoid cannot be visualized, but alignment appears to be normal. Compare this film with the transscapular view of the same patient shown in Figure 9-40.

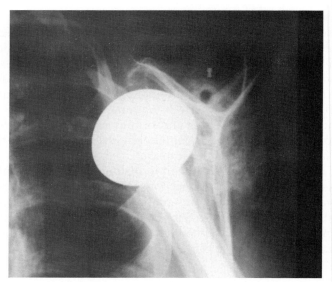

Figure 9-40. ▪ A transscapular view of the shoulder following arthroplasty. Note the coracoid and acromion processes and their intersection with the scapular spine, representing the glenoid fossa, and forming a "peace" or Mercedes-Benz symbol. Note that the humeral head is not centered, indicating a dislocation of the prosthetic head.

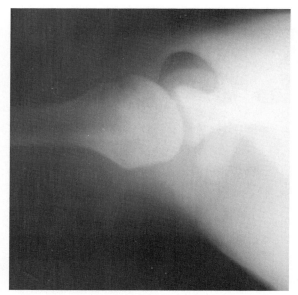

Figure 9-41. ▪ This axillary view demonstrates the alignment of the humeral head on the glenoid fossa. The acromion is seen to curve above the glenoid, and the coracoid points inferiorly.

Alignment

Normal alignment. Normal alignment for the West Point view will be through the glenohumeral joint

Abnormal alignment. Bankart lesion: A standard-routine series examined carefully for a Bankart lesion will usually rule out a history of complete dislocation if the trauma or event occurred more than 6 months before the examination. The Bankart lesion is the development of an osteophyte or periosteal reaction at the anterior inferior edge of the glenoid from the scuffing of the periosteum and bony edge of the glenoid by the passage of the humeral head over this edge in an anteroinferior dislocation. It can be described as a Bankart fracture when it includes a visible fracture of the anterior aspect of the inferior portion of the glenoid. Keep in mind that for the humeral head to dislocate from the glenohumeral joint, it must tear the glenoid labrum. The term "Bankart lesion" can also refer to the tear of the labrum, however, the torn labrum will not be demonstrated on standard x-ray examination but the effect of the dislocation on the bone is most often visible.

AC Joint

AP View

Alignment

Normal alignment. The distal clavicle will align with the acromion in a superior/inferior (coronal) plane. The AC joint should be less than 6 mm wide, and the injured side should have less than 50% greater width than the uninjured side. The coracoclavicular distance should be less than 11 mm or less than 50% more than the uninjured side.

Abnormal alignment. If the distal clavicle is not aligned with the acromion and the patient has sustained a fall onto the acromion, further imaging may be indicated. AC injuries normally are the result of trauma: a fall onto the shoulder, a collision with another person in sports, motor vehicle accidents, etc. Trauma can certainly be a predisposing factor for degenerative joint disease (DJD). Repetitive motion can damage this joint under the appropriate circumstances.

Bone

Normal bone. Check the distal end of the clavicle for fracture or arthritic changes.

Abnormal bone. Evaluate for clavicular fractures, displacement of the clavicle from the acromion articulating surface, arthritic changes of the AC joint, and cystic changes in the distal clavicle. (See Figure 9-42, and compare with Figure 9-8).

Cartilage. Cartilage is not evaluated in this view. The space between the distal clavicle and the acromion contains a fibrocartilaginous disc that is not visible on plain x-rays.

Soft tissue. Soft tissue is not evaluated in this view.

Test your understanding by taking a quiz on this chapter.

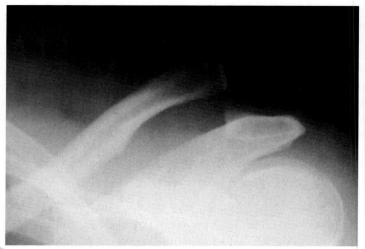

Figure **9-42.** ■ This AP view of the AC joint demonstrates a complete disruption of the AC joint with widening of the coracoclavicular space.

CASE STUDIES

Three case studies will now be presented. After reading the history and physical examination information, determine a PT diagnosis and design a treatment program. Look at the accompanying x-ray films. Use the ABCS system to evaluate the films. Do the x-ray films give you any additional information useful for treatment or prognosis?

CASE STUDY A

History: The patient is a 70-year-old female who fell from the back of a truck 10 years ago, fracturing her shoulder. She later had a total shoulder arthroplasty. She has just been to see her physician who has noted marked immobility in her shoulder. She has been referred to PT for shoulder ROM exercises.

In the first 2 weeks, she has made rapid progress and is now able to abduct to 90°, but is unable to improve beyond that. Her x-ray films are shown below.

Imaging:

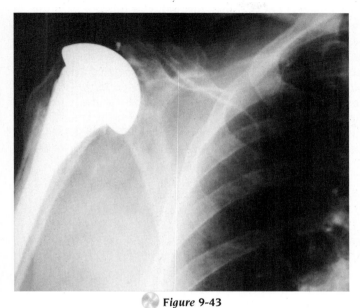

Figure 9-43

Images: Figures 9-43 and 9-44

Your impressions:

1. Alignment
2. Bone density and dimension
3. Cartilage
4. Soft tissue

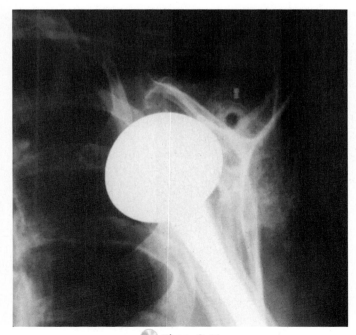

Figure 9-44

Our impressions:

When assessing a TSA, because the joint has been painful for so long before the surgery and the joint now has significantly reduced proprioception this means that the patient may be unaware of the joint's instability or frank dislocation. In this situation, a lateral scapular, or transscapular, view may be extremely revealing. The AP does not clearly demonstrate that this shoulder is dislocated, and the patient was not aware that it was dislocated and had been for some time. The clinical indication was that the patient could not progress beyond about 90° of forward flexion in spite of intensive PT. The shoulder had been in this condition for more than 10 years. The patient's pain was minimal, and she made excellent initial progress in therapy until she plateaued at 90°. Note on the transscapular view that the humerus is anterior to the holes that anchor the invisible glenoid portion of the prosthesis to the glenoid just above and below the intersection of the "Y" created by the lateral projection of the scapula.

Therapy questions:

A. How does this x-ray film alter your treatment program?

B. If this patient had just recently had her arthroplasty, would that change the treatment program?

C. What ROM is necessary for her to be functional?

CASE STUDY B

History: It is 2 weeks after the fracture, and the patient arrives in the clinic with a referral requesting "PT, evaluate and treat, 3 × week for 3 weeks."

Physical Findings: None at this time

Imaging:

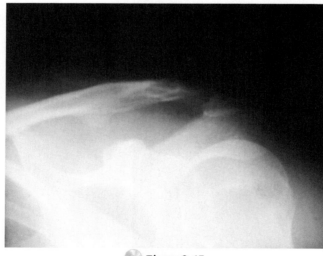

Figure 9-45

Image: Figure 9-45 Evaluate the AC joint for cystic and or degenerative changes and evidence of a fracture or separation. Review the margins of the visible portions of the ribs and the scapula. Compare Figure 9-45 with a normal AC joint in Figure 9-46.

Your impressions:

1. Alignment
2. Bone density and dimension
3. Cartilage
4. Soft tissue

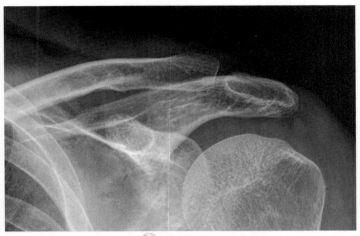

Figure 9-46

Our impressions:
1. Alignment: The clavicle is not aligned with the acromion. The coracoclavicular distance appears to be widened.
2. Bone density and dimension: There is a mottled appearance of the distal acromion, consistent with cystic changes of the clavicle.
3. Cartilage: Not applicable.
4. Soft tissue: Not applicable.

Therapy Questions:
A. How would you treat the patient in the clinic?
B. If this were an acute injury, at what time would you begin ROM and strengthening exercises?
C. Outline a program for optimizing shoulder function.

CASE STUDY C

History: This patient is a 37-year-old male who sustained a fracture of the inferior glenoid and dislocation during a fall from a treadmill in the gymnasium. The injury was a Bankart fracture that was surgically repaired. The week following surgery, the patient was sent to PT with a referral that gave the diagnosis, frequency, and duration of treatment and orders to "not let his shoulder get stiff." Please devise a treatment plan for this injury and compare it with a treatment you would have used for an impacted fracture of the surgical neck of the humerus.
Physical Findings: None at this time

Imaging:

Image: Figures 9-47 to 9-50

Your impressions:

1. Alignment
2. Bone density and dimension
3. Cartilage
4. Soft tissue

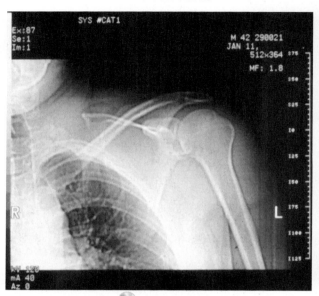

Figure 9-47

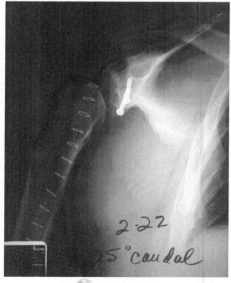

Figure 9-48

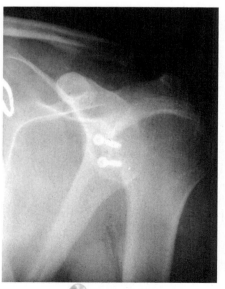

Figure 9-49

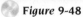

Figure 9-50

Our impressions (postsurgical views):
1. Alignment: The humeral head is aligned with the glenoid. There is a question as to whether the glenoid fragment is properly aligned with the glenoid.
2. Bone density and dimension: The bone density is consistent. The dimensions of the structures appear normal.
3. Cartilage: The cartilage space appears to be well maintained.
4. Soft tissue: Not applicable.

Therapy Questions:
A. What do the films tell you that you did not already know?
B. What will you do initially?
C. What will you wait on for 6 weeks after seeing the films?

REFERENCES

1. Resnick D, Niwayama G: *Diagnosis of bone and joint disorders,* ed 2, Philadelphia, 1998, WB Saunders.
2. McKinnis LN: *Fundamentals of orthopedic radiology,* Philadelphia, 1997, F.A. Davis.
3. Bernstein, J: Musculoskeletal Medicine, 1 ed, American Academy of Orthopaedic Surgeons, Rosemont, IL 2003, Page 243.
4. McKinnis LN: Diagnostic imaging of bones & joints. Plain-Film examination of the extremities, Home Study Course, 1999, Orthopedic Section of the APTA.
5. Greenspan A: *Orthopedic radiology,* ed 2, New York, 1992, Raven Press.

10 The Elbow, Wrist, and Hand

INTRODUCTION

Remarks

The hand and wrist are remarkable, from an engineering perspective, in their design, versatility, and function. They facilitate our abilities as "tool users" from rudimentary levers, wheels, and wedges to complex musical and medical instruments. They are exploratory instruments in dark and/or confined spaces, and they are used as shields when we are physically threatened (Figures 10-1 to 10-3). It is important when evaluating the hand, wrist, and elbow to understand that the functional muscle structure in the hand is for delicate manipulation relative to the strength provided by the extrinsic muscles within

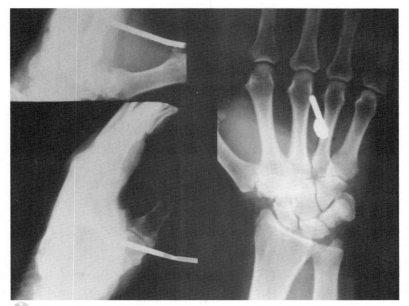

Figure 10-1. ■ A 75-year-old male tripped on sidewalk while walking and writing and fell onto his ballpoint pen creating a "stigmata"-type wound.

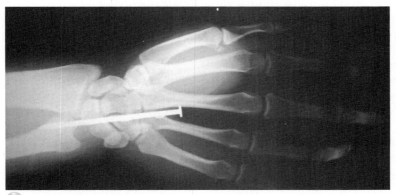

Figure 10-2. ■ A 27-year-old male carpenter tested his pneumatic nail gun by holding two of the "safety grips" and trigger while pressing his hand against the other safety on the barrel resulting in an almost "functional position" nailing of his carpals to his radius.

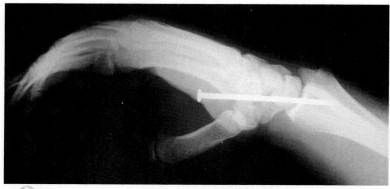

Figure 10-3. ■ Another view of same carpenter in Figure 10-2.

the forearm that power the distal joints of the digits. There are no intrinsic muscles of the fingers beyond the metacarpal phalangeal joints (MCPs) or within the carpals. The phalanges are moved into extension and flexion by a dorsal hood mechanism and volar flexor forearm muscles via pulley mechanisms respectively.

The elbow is the link between the shoulder and the carpals. It allows flexion and extension and supination and pronation via an articulation, or hinge, between the distal humerus and the ulna and supination and pronation via the radial head and the capitellum.

Another useful construct is to view the carpals as a proximal row made up, from radial to ulnar, of the scaphoid, lunate, and triquetrum and a distal row made up of the trapezium (the trapeze that the thumb swings on), trapezoid, capitate, and hamate. The pisiform is largely regarded as a sesamoid bone within the flexor carpi ulnaris tendon. The integrity of the wrist is maintained by the extensive investment of the carpal ligaments. Stretching and/or damaging these ligaments results in the malalignment of the carpal bones. The bones depend upon the support of the ligaments and the other carpals for their stability. For example, the capitate alone articulates and is supported by at least eight other bones. If this support is compromised by a damaged ligament or bone, as when a scaphoid is fractured and collapses or the scapholunate ligament is torn or stretched, the delicate balance that is the wrist will shift, and multiple malalignments will ensue.

OBJECTIVES

1. Recall the three standard elbow views, three standard wrist views, three standard hand views, two standard thumb views, and the phalanges view and their purposes.
2. Identify the normal and pathologic alignment of the standard views of the elbow, wrist, and hand.
3. Identify the normal and pathologic dimensions and densities of the elbow, wrist, and hand bones.
4. Identify normal and pathologic cartilage.
5. Identify the normal and pathologic presentation of soft tissue.
6. Identify film abnormalities, given a history and x-ray film.
7. Use x-ray film information to adjust a physical therapy treatment program.

STANDARD VIEWS

Hand

The hand is evaluated with a posteroanterior (PA), a lateral, and an oblique view (Figures 10-4 to 10-6).

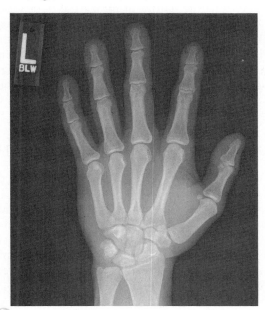

Figure 10-4. ■ An anterior to posterior view of a normal hand and wrist.

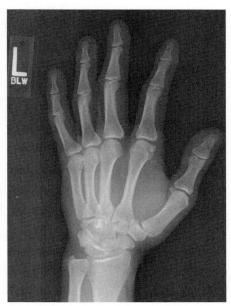

Figure 10-5. ■ An oblique view of a normal hand and wrist.

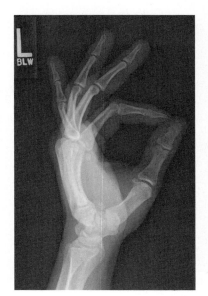

Figure 10-6. ■ A lateral view of a normal hand and wrist.

Wrist

The standard views of the wrist are a PA, lateral, and a semipronated oblique. X-ray examination of the wrist is the most important tool for diagnosis of fractures and dislocations of the wrist and the PA and lateral views provide the most useful view.[1] The semipronated oblique allows the evaluation of the scaphoid and the distal radius.[2] The dynamic nature of the carpal bones that accompanies movements in the wrist and hand requires multiple other views to emphasize and evaluate the slight changes that occur in the alignment of the carpals. Special views may include radial and ulnar deviation, which is helpful to visualize the carpals and specifically the scaphoid when in ulnar deviation, semisupinated oblique, dorsal and palmar flexion, scaphoid, and carpal tunnel views.

Digits

The standard views of the fingers are the lateral, PA and oblique views.[3] (Figures 10-7 to 10-9).

Elbow

The standard views of the elbow are the anteroposterior (AP) with the hand supinated, the lateral with the hand positioned laterally, and the oblique with the hand pronated.[4] A special view to include the olecranon, the flexion view, is taken with the elbow fully flexed, and the beam enters the distal forearm and progresses through the distal humerus and radial head views, taken in supination and pronation to allow assessment of the radial head (Figures 10-10 to 10-12).

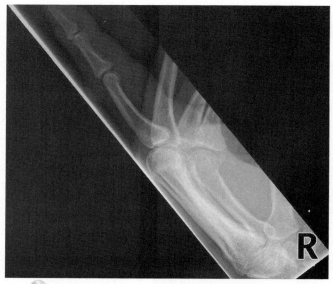

Figure 10-7. ■ A lateral view of a normal digit.

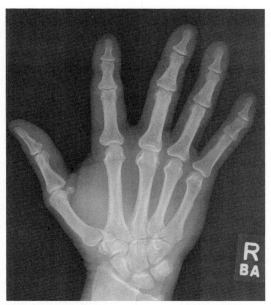

Figure 10-8. ■ A PA view of a normal hand and wrist and lateral view of a normal thumb.

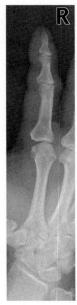

Figure 10-9. ■ An oblique view of a normal first digit.

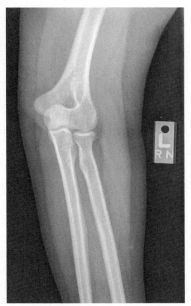

Figure 10-10. ■ An oblique view of a normal elbow.

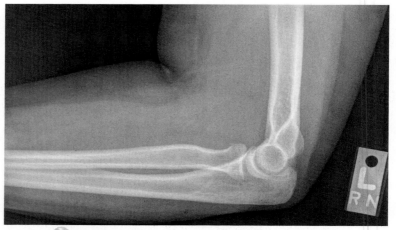

Figure 10-11. ■ A lateral view of a normal elbow.

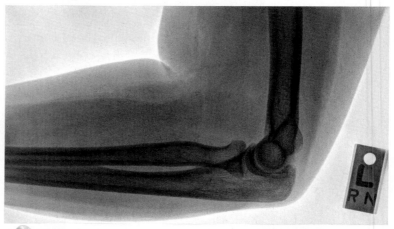

Figure 10-12. ■ A contrast color lateral view of a normal elbow.

EVALUATION OF THE ELBOW, WRIST, AND HAND USING ABCS

Elbow AP

Alignment

Normal alignment. It is best to begin the evaluation by carefully identifying the following structures on the AP view from proximal to distal: the olecranon fossa, the medial humeral epicondyle, the lateral humeral epicondyles, the olecranon, trochlea, capitellum, coronoid process, and the radial head (Figure 10-13). The AP, lateral, and oblique views mentioned earlier must demonstrate that the radial head is aligned with, but not in contact with, the capitellum. The

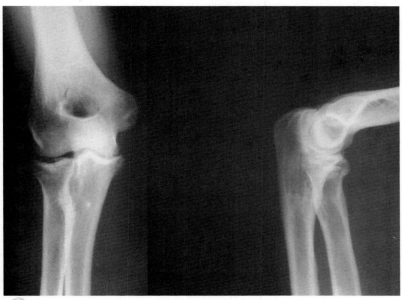

Figure 10-13. ■ An oblique view on the left and a lateral view demonstrating the olecranon fossa, the medial humeral epicondyle, the lateral humeral epicondyles, the olecranon, trochlea, capitellum, coronoid process, and the radial head.

olecranon should be centered on the olecranon fossa in the AP view. The "carrying angle," a valgus angle demonstrated by a line drawn down the center of the humerus that intersects a line drawn up through the center of the ulna, should be about 15 degrees.[5]

Abnormal. Any evidence of a malalignment between the olecranon and its fossa, particularly in the lateral view, must be carefully evaluated. In one case, an individual sought help from an orthopedic surgeon after months of suffering with a dislocated elbow that had been "reduced" by a chiropractor.[6] Children are particularly prone to dislocations of the elbow as a result of their activities and immature bone structure (Figures 10-14 to 10-16).

Figures 10-17 and 10-18 are lateral and oblique views of a young man with a dislocated elbow.

Bone Density and Dimension

Normal. The radial head should be carefully evaluated for any evidence of bone chips or fractures. The medial and lateral epicondyles of the distal humerus must be evaluated for any lucencies or breaks in the margins (Figure 10-19).

Abnormal. Radial head fractures can be difficult to recognize, particularly if they are nondisplaced. If there is evidence of swelling or occult bleeding (see "sail sign" under "Soft Tissue" later), the patient may need a CT or an MRI to definitively diagnose the injury. There are three types of radial head

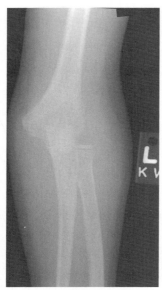

Figure 10-14. ■ An AP view of a dislocated left elbow in a 10-year-old male.

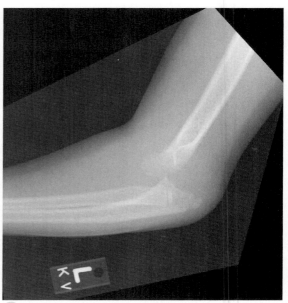

Figure 10-15. ■ A lateral view of a dislocated left elbow in a 10-year-old male.

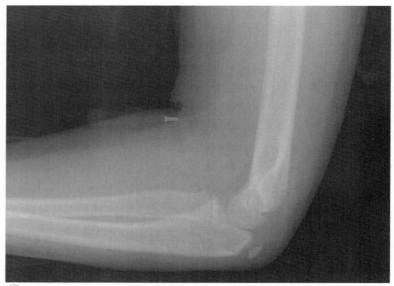

Figure 10-16. ■ A lateral view of reduced dislocated elbow in a 10-year-old male who was wrestling with his older brother and sustained a dislocated left elbow.

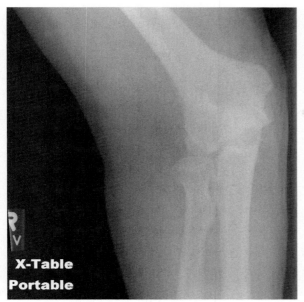

Figure 10-17. ■ Note the "markedly increased angle between the ulna and the humerus at the olecranon and the displacement of the radial head relative to the capitellum."

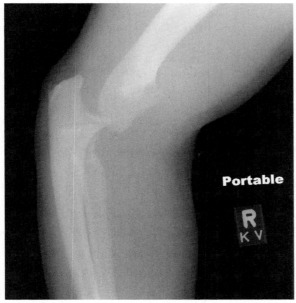

Figure 10-18. ■ A lateral view of the dislocated elbow seen in Figure 10-17.

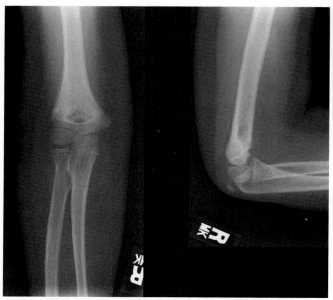

Figure 10-19. ■ Lateral and AP views of the elbow reveal a supra-condylar fracture in this skeletally immature individual.

fractures: type I are nondisplaced, type II fractures are displaced, and type III are comminuted.[7,8]

Cartilage

Normal. Cartilage is usually evaluated in the elbow with an MRI. Osteo-chondritis dissecans can be diagnosed with MRI or CT.

Abnormal. Damage to the cartilage in the elbow can be from trauma, infection, systemic disease, as in rheumatoid arthritis, trauma, or heavy repetitive use. It is diagnosed with clinical examination, arthrography and CT.[9]

Soft Tissue

Normal. The lateral view demonstrates soft tissue anterior and posterior to the distal humerus that is consistent and without decreased density.

Abnormal. If there is an occult fracture of the radial head or epicondyle(s), the soft tissue and/or fat pad is elevated from the periosteum by the bleeding and is identified as an area of decreased density, usually anterior to the distal humerus. This was thought to resemble a sail on a boat. This is evidence of bleeding or swelling and is known as a "sail sign" or "fat pad sign" and at a minimum requires further work-up to rule out a fracture.[10] (Figure 10-20)

Elbow Lateral

Alignment

Normal. The lateral view is taken with the arm abducted and the hand in neutral rotation. The structures to be identified are the overlapping trochlea and the capitellum and the overlapping radial head and the coronoid process

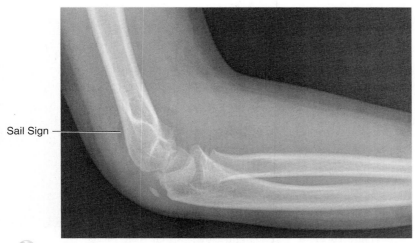

Sail Sign

Figure 10-20. ■ On this lateral view, the "sail sign" is more evident posteriorly than anteriorly, but both are visible with close inspection.

(Figure 10-21). A line drawn down the center of the humeral shaft should intersect a line drawn through the center of the shaft of the radius at approximately 90 degrees.

Abnormal. As noted earlier, the lateral view is the most sensitive to dislocations and/or subluxations. In children a line drawn down the anterior shaft of the humerus will intersect the capitellum (a separate center of ossification in children). A line drawn along the shaft of the radius will intersect the line from the humerus in the capitellum. A variation in this intersection, as is found on Figure 10-23, indicates a potential fracture in the supracondylar region of the humerus or dislocation of the elbow joint. (Figures 10-22 and 10-23).

Bone Density and Dimension

The elbow is evaluated for changes in the bone density with particular attention paid to the radial head. When evaluating a patient for a fracture of the ulna, always look for an accompanying dislocation of the radial head known as a "Monteggia's fracture-dislocation." This radial head displacement may be subtle and requires careful evaluation (Figures 10-24 to 10-26).

Cartilage

Normal. The joint space is well maintained, and the articular surfaces are smooth and without osteophytes or decreased densities.

Abnormal. The joint spaces are markedly decreased or absent, there may be osteophytosis and, if severe, angulation of the joint from chronic erosion of the joint accompanied by increased bone density around the articular surfaces (Figures 10-27 and 10-28).

Soft Tissue

Normal. The soft tissue is carefully evaluated along the metaphysis of the bone for changes in density (Figure 10-29).

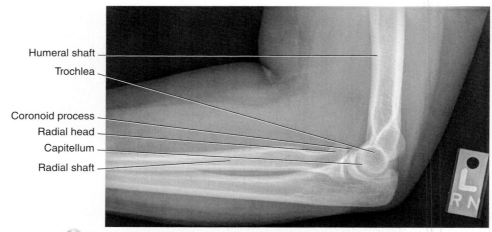

Humeral shaft
Trochlea
Coronoid process
Radial head
Capitellum
Radial shaft

Figure 10-21. ■ x-ray, lateral view, normal

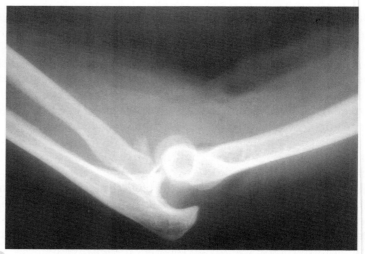

Figure 10-22. ■ Clearly the olecranon is posterior to the humeral olecranon fossa.

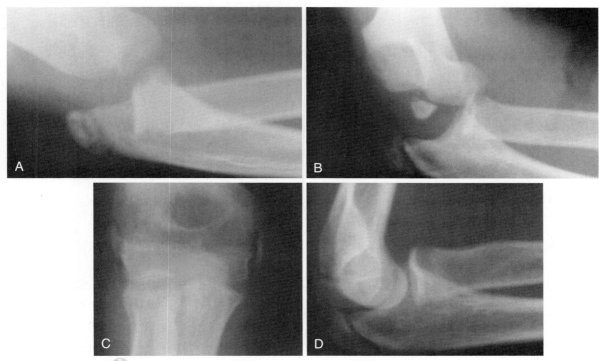

Figure 10-23. ■ Dislocation of elbow and fracture of radial head. **A.** Posterior dislocation of elbow with suggestion of osteochondral fragment from radial head fracture. **B.** Oblique radiograph shows loose fragments of radial head entrapped within joint. **C and D.** After open reduction and excision of loose fragment. Obvious ossification around both collateral ligaments and callus in area of radial head and neck are seen in **C.** *(From Canale ST, Beaty JH: Campbell's Operative Orthopedics, 11e, St. Louis, Mosby, 2007.)*

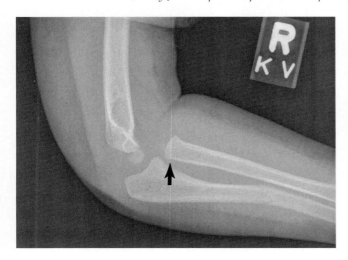

Figure 10-24. ■ A lateral view of a child's elbow with a Monteggia's fracture-dislocation of the ulna and radial head.

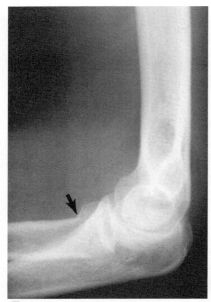

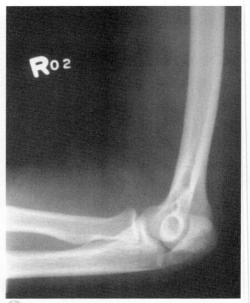

Figure 10-25. ■ Radial head fracture on lateral view; note *arrow.*

Figure 10-26. ■ Olecranon fracture on lateral view.

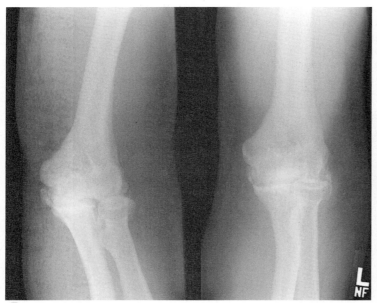

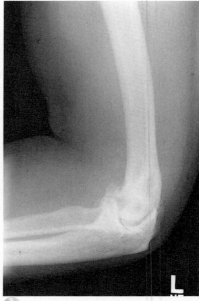

Figure 10-27. ■ AP and oblique views of an elbow with severe osteoarthritic changes.

Figure 10-28. ■ A lateral view of the same individual's elbow as seen in Figure 10-27.

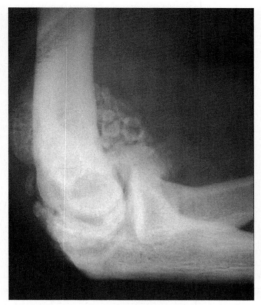

Figure 10-29. ■ An osteochondroma, seen in a lateral elbow view.

Abnormal. Changes in density may indicate elevation of the fat pad or the periosteal soft tissue by bleeding or swelling from an occult, non-displaced fracture of the joint or the radial head. It can appear more pronounced just proximal to the joint and less so more proximally along the diaphysis of the humerus. This is referred to as the "sail sign" or "fat pad sign" [10] (Figure 10-30).

Wrist PA

Alignment

Normal. Begin the initial evaluation by identifying the bones of the wrist and their relative positions to one another based upon the type of view that is evaluated. For purposes of evaluation the wrist is comprised of the distal radius and ulna, the proximal row of carpals, the distal row of carpals and the proximal metacarpals.[11] The carpals articulate with the distal radius, the other carpals and, distally the base of the metacarpals. The dorsal and volar surfaces serve as attachment sites for the carpal ligaments that are critical for maintaining the delicate articular relationships of the bones of the wrist.[12] For normal views of the wrist, see Figures 10-4, 10-5, and 10-6.

Abnormal

1. Colles' fracture (Figure 10-31) and Smith's fracture (Figure 10-32) are common examples of fractures of the wrist.
2. Carpal instabilities

Scapholunate dissociation (See Figure 10-34): This is the most common form of

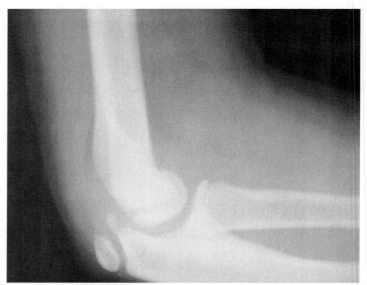

Figure 10-30. ■ A lateral view of the elbow with a "sail sign" or "fat pad sign" in this child, indicating an occult fracture of the distal humerus.

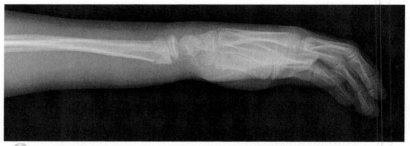

Figure 10-31. ■ A lateral view of the wrist demonstrating a fracture of the distal radius with slight dorsal angulation, which is a Colles' fracture.

carpal instability and is the result of damage or tearing of the scapholunate ligament. The damage is diagnosed on the AP film by measuring the distance between the lunate and the proximal scaphoid. If this distance is 3 mm or more, it is considered diagnostic of scapholunate dissociation.[13] This increased gap is also known as a "Terry Thomas" sign after the British comedian who had a significant gap between his two front teeth, hence the name. Untreated, this can progress to scaphoid erosion into the distal radius, creating a painful wrist or further carpal damage (Figures 10-33 and 10-34). If there is an old fracture of the scaphoid that has collapsed or a long-standing

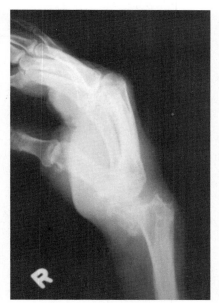

Figure 10-32. ■ A lateral view of the wrist demonstrating a fracture of the distal radius with volar angulation, which is a Smith's fracture.

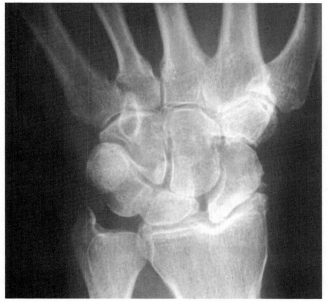

Figure 10-33. ■ A positive "Terry Thomas" sign and radial erosion.

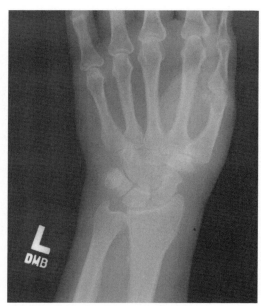

Figure 10-34. ■ An AP view of the wrist demonstrating scapholunate dissociation.

scapholunate dissociation, the scaphoid may rotate progressively into flexion and be viewed on an AP view as "on end" or along the long axis of the scaphoid. This presents itself as a scaphoid ring sign also called a "signet ring" sign. This is because when viewing the scaphoid along its axis on an AP view after the scaphoid has rotated or displaced, the "ring" is the long axis view of the cortical margins of the bone.[14] (If a piece of PVC pipe were x-rayed on an AP view, the margins would be more dense the way a tibia, femur, or humerus appears; however, if these same bones are rotated to x-ray them along their long axis [an axial view], they appear circular. This same concept applies to the unstable, rotated scaphoid.)

3. Scapholunate advanced collapse (SLAC)

   This is the result of a long-standing carpal instability; there is degeneration in the scaphoradial joint, and eventually the capitate subluxes onto the lunate dorsally (Figures 10-35 to 10-40).

   Bone Density and Dimension

   Normal. Normal bone should be uniform for the view that is evaluated. The hook of the hamate, for example, will appear as an increased density over the body of the bone, and the shape of the hook will be determined by the view that is evaluated.

   Abnormal. Bones of the wrist (carpals) and hand should be carefully evaluated after trauma for the most common fractures, specifically fractures of the scaphoid, the most commonly fractured bone of the wrist. Commonly injured by a fall on an outstretched hand, it may be difficult to visualize on

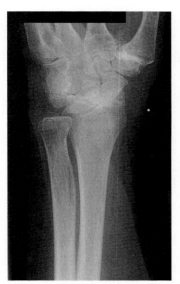

Figure 10-35. ■ Note on zoom-in-view the cystic formation of the distal radius indicative of advanced OA and the "whitening" of the bone, also called "eburnation," at the scaphoid distal radial joint. The eburnation is a result of "bone-on-bone" articulation indicating that all of the hyaline cartilage has been destroyed. Oblique view of the wrist showing cystic formation at the radial scaphoid joint.

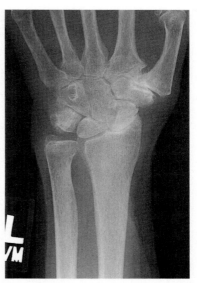

Figure 10-36. ■ An AP view of the wrist showing cystic formation at the radial scaphoid joint.

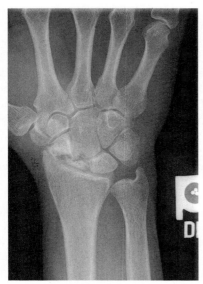

Figure 10-37. ■ An AP view of the wrist showing an old scaphoid fracture with collapse of the scaphoid.

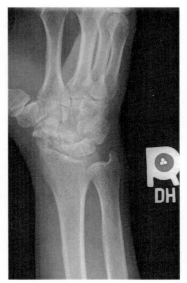

Figure 10-38. ■ An oblique view of the wrist showing an old scaphoid fracture with collapse of the scaphoid in the same individual seen in Figure 10-37.

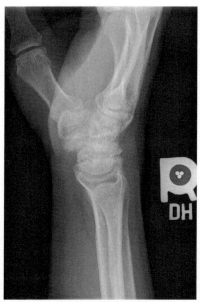

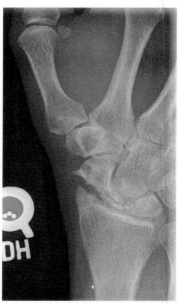

Figure 10-39. ■ A lateral view of the wrist showing an old scaphoid fracture with collapse of the scaphoid in the same individual seen in Figure 10-37.

Figure 10-40. ■ An oblique tomogram view of the wrist showing an old scaphoid fracture with collapse of the scaphoid in the same individual seen in Figure 10-37.

plain films for the first few weeks. Any patient having sustained a fall onto an outstretched hand with tenderness and swelling in the anatomic snuff box is clinically presumed to have a fractured scaphoid until proven otherwise. If not properly treated early, this fracture has a relatively high rate of non-union or delayed union. A bone scan or CT can be extremely helpful when in doubt and a decision is required for immediate purposes (e.g., can a soldier be scheduled for deployment to accompany his unit overseas, or can an athlete compete in the "big game" or track meet?) A bone scan will be positive within 24 to 48 hours, and a CT or MRI, although considerably more expensive than a bone scan, may also provide immediate confirmation (Figures 10-41 to 10-44).

Cartilage

Normal. The joint space will be equal between the carpals with no evidence of bone-on-bone erosion.

Abnormal. As a result of a fracture or carpal instability, there may be a malalignment of one or more of the carpals, and if the problem is of long-standing duration, there may be erosion and whitening, or eburnation, of the bones where they are in contact (Figures 10-45 to 10-47).

Soft Tissue

Normal. Between the distal ulna, the distal radius, and the proximal triquetrum is a fibrocartilaginous "articular disc" that is not visible on plain films and must be evaluated by MRI or injection with a dye before imaging.

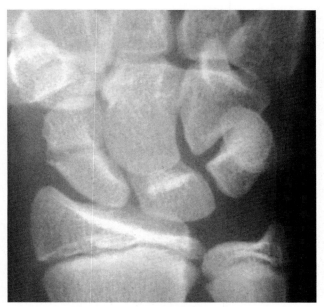

Figure 10-41. ■ An obvious fracture and displacement of the scaphoid in a skeletally immature individual.

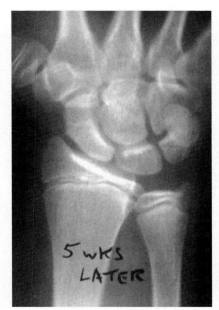

Figure 10-42. ■ The same individual as Figure 10-41, 5 weeks later after immobilization. Fracture demonstrates acceptable healing for this date after injury.

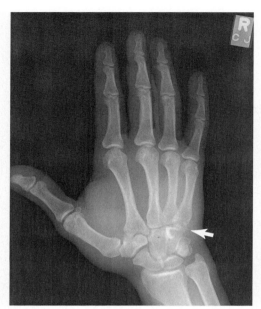

Figure **10-43.** ■ Oblique view of a fracture of the hamate bone. Note: The fracture is very subtle and requires magnification of this film to demonstrate fracture.

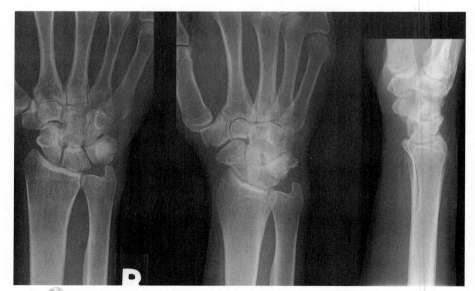

Figure **10-44.** ■ Three views, P/A, Oblique and lateral of the wrist demonstrating DJD of the Capitate demonstrating carpal collapse and cystic formation.

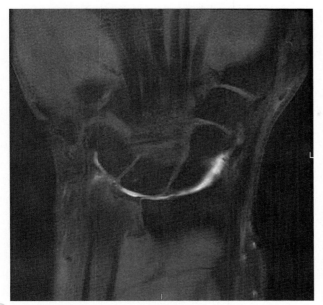

Figure 10-45. ■ MRI, T2, of the proximal row of the carpals.

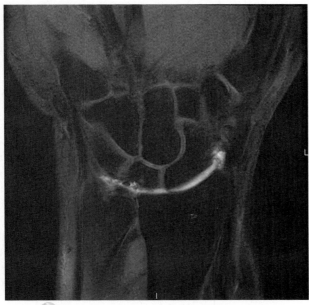

Figure 10-46. ■ MRI, T2, of the carpals.

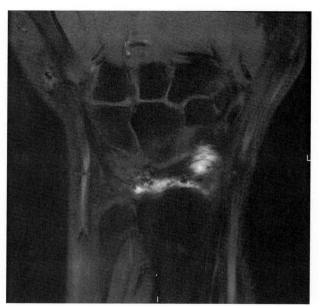

Figure 10-47. ■ MRI, T2, of the carpals. Note the loose bodies *(dark dots)* in the dorsal radial carpal space.

Wrist Lateral

Alignment

Normal. (See Figure 10-44 right) The lateral view demonstrates the alignment of, proximal to distal, the distal radius, the lunate, the capitate and the metacarpal of the third (long) finger. All of these bones should fall in the longitudinal line drawn through the center of the third finger.[15]

Displacement of the lunate dorsally or volarly with rotation is indicative of scapholunate dissociations/instability as a result of previous carpal damage and/or ligamentous damage.

On the normal lateral view, a line drawn proximal to distal through the center of the radius and the third metacarpal should intersect the centers of the lunate and the capitate. The distal radius is normally angled toward the ulna at an angle of 15 to 25 degrees and has a palmar angulation of about the same angle. The distal radius articulates with the scaphoid and the lunate carpal bones and has concavities that reflect these articular surfaces, but they are not visible on the plain films. In scapholunate dissociation, the lateral view may be evaluated by drawing the following lines: (1) a line through the middle of the long axis of the scaphoid and (2) a line perpendicular to the long axis at the midpoint of the lunate. The angle that is formed proximally by the intersection of these two lines is measured and should be 30 to 60 degrees. An increase in this angle of greater than 20 degrees indicates increased scaphoid flexion and/or lunate extension or both and suggests carpal instability.[16]

Abnormal. (Note: The examples that follow have lateral and PA views together to allow better visualization of the structures.)

Bone Density and Dimension

Normal. The carpal and metacarpal bones will overlap on the lateral view, and the alignment as discussed previously is critical. The bones should be identified and the margins carefully traced for lucencies and changes in density that may indicate early avascular necrosis of a fractured scaphoid or lunate (Kienböck's disease, Figure 10-48). Kienböck's disease, or avascular necrosis of the lunate carpal, is identified by a progressive increasing density on plain films of the lunate, when compared with the healthy bones adjacent to the lunate. Eventually the bone may undergo cystic degeneration and eventual collapse accompanied by gradual collapse of the proximal row of the carpals.[17]

Abnormal. A fracture at the junction of the diaphysis and the metaphysis in the forearm is referred to as a 'buckle' or torus fracture (See Figure 10-51).[18] The lateral view will demonstrate the dorsal (Colles') or volar/palmar, angulation

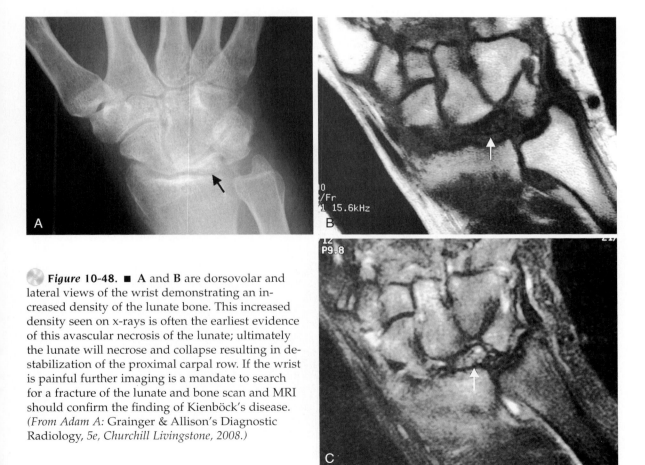

Figure 10-48. ■ A and B are dorsovolar and lateral views of the wrist demonstrating an increased density of the lunate bone. This increased density seen on x-rays is often the earliest evidence of this avascular necrosis of the lunate; ultimately the lunate will necrose and collapse resulting in destabilization of the proximal carpal row. If the wrist is painful further imaging is a mandate to search for a fracture of the lunate and bone scan and MRI should confirm the finding of Kienböck's disease. *(From Adam A:* Grainger & Allison's Diagnostic Radiology, *5e, Churchill Livingstone, 2008.)*

(Smith's) of fractures of the distal radius (Figures 10-49 and 10-50). A fracture of the metaphysis of the distal radius may compress, collapse, or telescope and appear on the AP as angulated radially or ulnarly and on the lateral view as angled in a dorsal or palmar direction. If the diagnosis is in question, comparison views of the opposite distal radius are extremely helpful (Figures 10-51 to 10-53).

Cartilage and soft tissue are not evaluated on the lateral projection of the wrist.

Wrist Oblique

The oblique view of the wrist will sometimes demonstrate a better view of the hand and wrist, exposing fractures, malalignments, and instabilities not seen on the AP and lateral views. There are multiple oblique views accompanying the series shown previously (see Figures 10-51 and 10-53).

ABC review for the wrist oblique view is not necessary.

Hand and Distal Radial Fractures and Metacarpal Injuries PA, Lateral, and Oblique

The standard views of the hand are: PA, oblique, and lateral.[19]
Alignment
Normal. The P/A view demonstrates an ulna and radius that align distally. This alignment constitutes a "neutral ulnar variance." The distal radius should not contact any of the carpals but its palmar angulation and concavities for

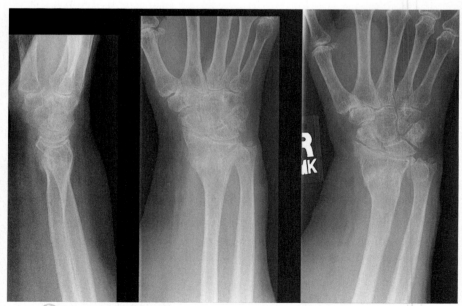

Figure 10-49. ■ Three views, lateral, oblique and P/A of the wrist demonstrating a fracture of the distal radius.

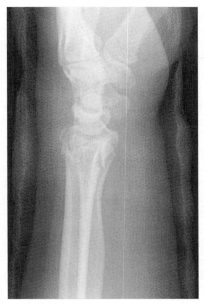

Figure 10-50. ■ Lateral view of a casted distal radial fracture.

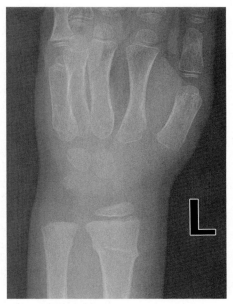

Figure 10-51. ■ Oblique view, 5-year-old male, buckle fracture of radius.

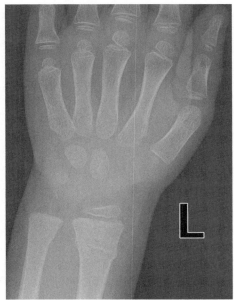

Figure 10-52. ■ A/P view, 5-year-old male, buckle fx.

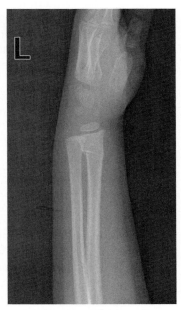

Figure 10-53. ■ Lateral view, 5-year-old male, buckle fx. Note the dorsal angulation of the distal radial component.

articulation with the scaphoid and lunate give the appearance on this view of a slight overlap. The distal radius is normally angled toward the ulna at an angle of 15 to 25 degrees and has a palmar angulation of about the same angle. The distal radius articulates with the scaphoid and the lunate carpal bones and has concavities that reflect these articular surfaces, but the concavities are not visible on the plain films.

Abnormal. If the ulna does not project far enough distally to align with the radius, that is a "negative ulnar variance," and if the ulna projects distally past the ulnar margin of the radius, it is a "positive ulnar variance."[20]

The Colles' fracture, the most common fracture of the distal radius, is a dorsal angulation and displacement with radial angulation of the distal fragment of a fracture of the distal radius.[21] A Smith's fracture is a palmar/volar, angulation of the distal radial fragment when the distal radius is fractured. These fractures are best assessed on the lateral view, but the PA and oblique views may demonstrate impaction of the distal fragment into the radius (a bayonet-shaped deformity) and radial or ulnar displacement resulting in shortening of the radius. The lateral view will demonstrate the dorsal (Colles') or volar/palmar angulation (Smith's) of any fractures of the distal radius (Figures 10-54 and 10-55).

Bone Density and Dimension
Normal. The metacarpal bones of the hand should be without a malalignment or evidence of decreased density that may represent a fracture. These bones should, except for length, be similar in shape, and the adjacent bones may sometimes be used for comparison. If a fracture is identified or suspected, additional PA, lateral, and oblique views may be necessary to define the extent and comminution components of the fracture or tumor.

Abnormal. The distal radius is the most commonly fractured bone of the distal arm (Figures 10-56 to 10-85).

Cartilage
Normal and abnormal evaluation of the cartilage is as covered previously in this chapter (Figures 10-86 to 10-88).

Phalanges PA and Lateral

Alignment
Normal. The PA view of the fingers should demonstrate the joint spaces of the interphalangeal joints (IPs) that are equally well maintained and aligned along a line drawn through the middle of the bones along their long axis. The lateral view provides the opportunity to isolate the lateral projection of one or more of the phalanges through positioning of the hand. The digit of interest is flexed sufficiently to bring it out of alignment with the other digits.

Abnormal. Fractures are normally the result of trauma. Remember that the phalanges are small bones on the ends of our hands with little or no soft tissue protection. They can be cut, crushed, twisted, hammered, etc. Examine Figures 10-89 to 10-93 and look for evidence of bony injury.

Rheumatoid arthritis destroys connective tissue. As joints are destroyed, they are prone to a malalignment with erosion of the joint spaces, ulnar drift of the

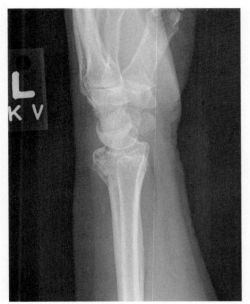

Figure 10-54. ■ Lateral view, acute distal, comminuted radius fracture with dorsal angulation (Colles' fracture).

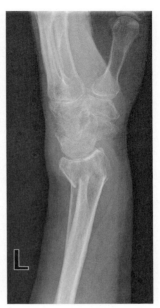

Figure 10-55. ■ Lateral view, acute distal, radial fx, comminuted with dorsal displacement (Colles' fracture).

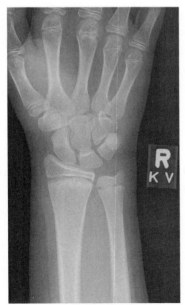

Figure 10-56. ■ P/A view of a Salter-Harris II fracture of the distal radius. Note: The fracture is not visualized on this view.

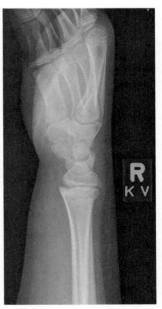

Figure 10-57. ■ Lateral view of a Salter-Harris II fracture of the distal radius. This view demonstrates that the fragment is buckled and displaced dorsally.

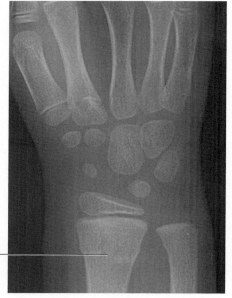

Greenstick fracture

Figure 10-58. ■ P/A view of a 'greenstick fracture' of the radius in a 5-year-old.

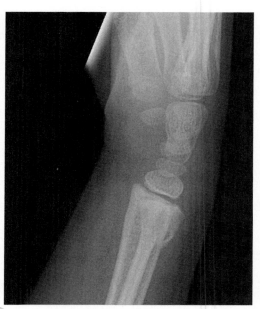

Figure 10-59. ■ Note that a greenstick fracture occurs in skeletally immature individuals when the bone is soft enough or not mineralized enough to allow one side, in this case the dorsal side, to buckle but the palmer-ventral side gives enough to prevent breaking, hence the name a "greenstick" fracture.

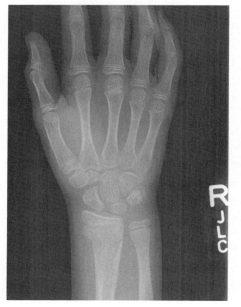

Figure 10-60. ■ P/A view of a Colles fracture in a child. Note the fracture line proximal to the distal growth plate.

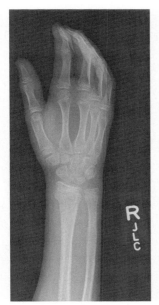

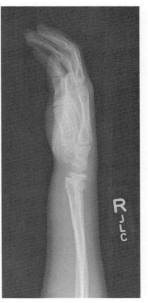

Figure 10-61. ■ Oblique view of a Colles fracture in a child.

Figure 10-62. ■ Lateral view of a Colles fracture in a child. Note the dorsal angulation of the distal fracture fragment.

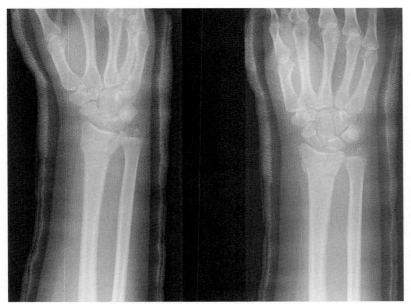

Figure 10-63. ■ P/A and oblique views of a comminuted fracture of the distal radius in a cast.

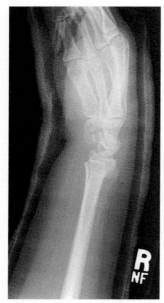

Figure 10-64. ■ This view shows the intraarticular component on one view only, the oblique view.

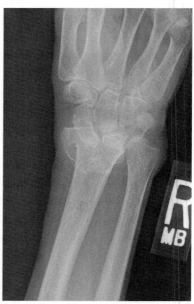

Figure 10-65. ■ P/A view, of an acute distal radial fracture with dorsal angulation.

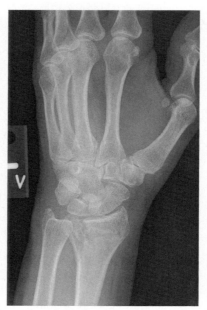

Figure 10-66. ■ Oblique view of an acute, intraarticular, distal radial fracture.

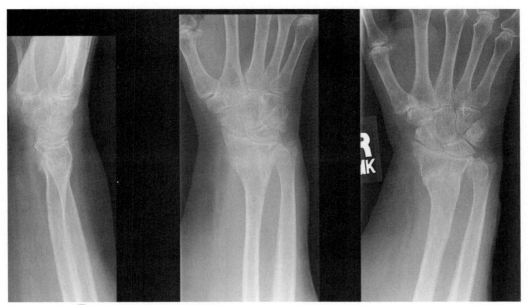

Figure 10-67. ■ Note that the comminution is not as readily apparent on the P/A view as on the oblique view, which demonstrates the intraarticular component of this fracture and the ulnar styloid fracture, and the lateral view demonstrates the dorsal angulation of this fracture. All three views are important.

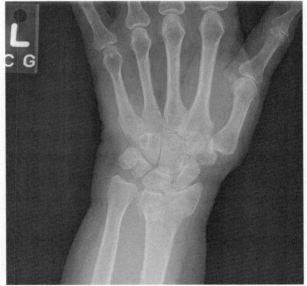

Figure 10-68. ■ P/A view of a comminuted intraarticular distal radial fracture.

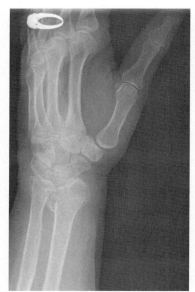

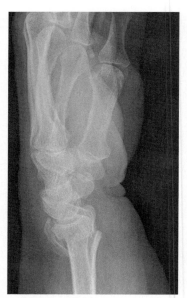

Figure 10-69. ■ Oblique view of comminuted, intraarticular fracture of the distal radius. Doral angulation is visible on this view. Demonstrates comminution and shortening of the radius and overlap of the distal fragments with proximal component of distal radius.

Figure 10-70. ■ Lateral view of a comminuted, intraarticular fracture of the distal radius. Dorsal angulation of the distal fragment is clear on this view.

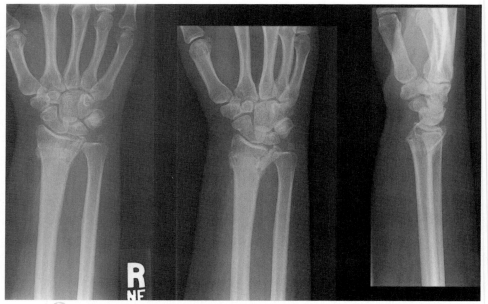

Figure 10-71. ■ Three view, P/A, Oblique, and lateral of a comminuted, intraarticular, distal radial fracture with dorsal angulation.

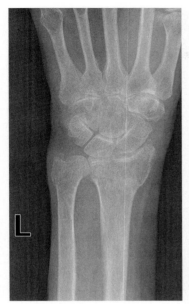

Figure 10-72. ■ Note shortening of radius accompanying this Colles' fracture.

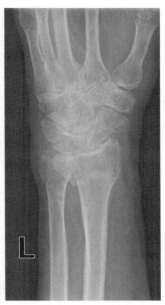

Figure 10-73. ■ Oblique view of a fracture of the distal radius and ulna with shortening.

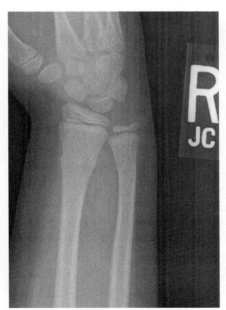

Figure 10-74. ■ Oblique view of a Buckle fracture in a child of the distal radius and ulna. Note the angulation and radial "bump" at the fracture site.

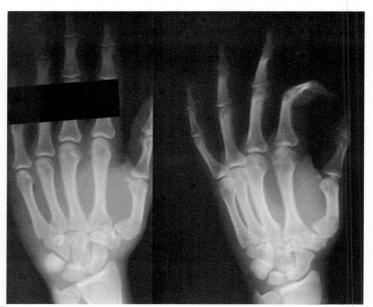

Figure 10-75. ■ A 23-year-old male with a fracture of the first metacarpal shaft proximally was casted and sent home and scheduled for follow-up. He returned 1 month later and had been noncompliant with hand protection. Follow-up x-ray (October 1999) demonstrated marked increase in angulation of fracture and showed no healing callus around fracture.

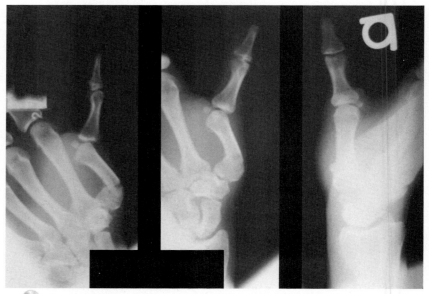

Figure 10-76. ■ Follow-up x-ray from Figure 10-75 demonstrated marked increase in angulation of fracture and showed no healing callus around fracture.

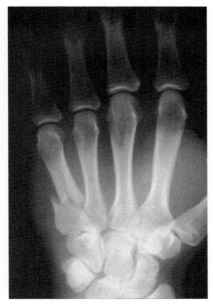

Figure 10-77. ■ Fracture of the base of the shaft of the fifth metacarpal, sometimes referred to as a "karate chop" fracture.

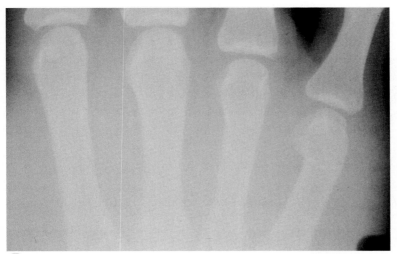

Figure 10-78. ■ "Boxer's fracture" of the distal fifth metacarpal shaft, also known as a "Dear John" fracture. These occur when the fisted hand forcefully strikes a firm, relatively unyielding surface, such as a wall, door, or a facial bone(s). The fracture may occur on the other metacarpals, but the fifth metacarpal is most often involved. This x-ray, although of poor quality, demonstrates rotation of the distal fragment.

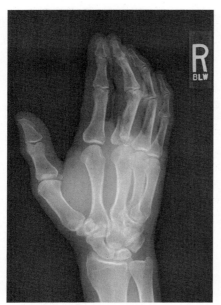

Figure 10-79. ■ Oblique view of an intraarticular fracture of the third proximal phalanx. This was done to an adult who was playing a game where the two opponents attempt to slide their hands out from under their opponents and make a fist and crack the opponent on the knuckles before the opponent can move his hands. If they miss completely, their opponent becomes the one who attempts to strike them.

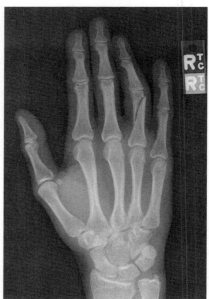

Figure 10-80. ■ P/A view of a fracture of the fourth proximal phalanx by an individual playing a game called 'Mercy' where one participant strikes the hand of another with fisted knuckles until they ask for "Mercy".

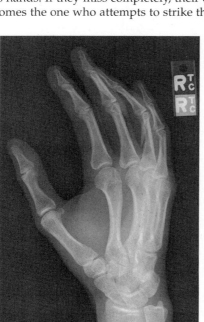

Figure 10-81. ■ Oblique view of the same injury as Figure 10-80.

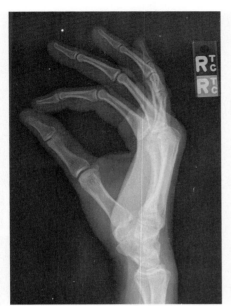

Figure 10-82. ■ Lateral view of the same injury as in Figure 10-80. The fracture, although easily seen on the AP and the oblique, is very difficult to see on the lateral.

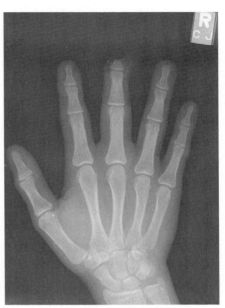

Figure 10-83. ■ P/A view of a partial amputation of the distal phalanx of the third finger.

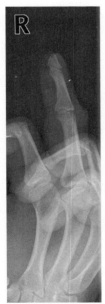

Figure 10-84. ■ Oblique view of a partial amputation of the distal phalanx of the third finger.

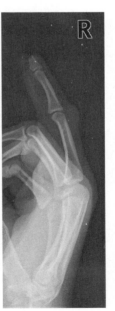

Figure 10-85. ■ Lateral view of a partial amputation of the distal phalanx of the third finger.

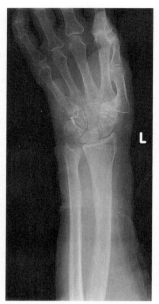

Figure 10-86. ■ P/A view of a hand with severe degenerative joint disease (DJD).

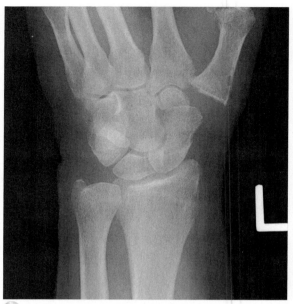

Figure 10-87. ■ Oblique view of the wrist trapezium absent.

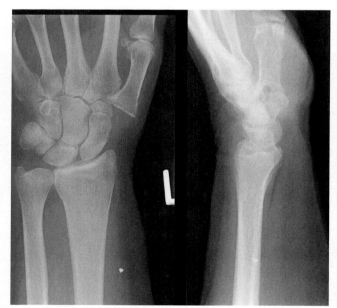

Figure 10-88. ■ The straight edge on the proximal first metacarpal (thumb) appears to be a result of surgical intervention and may explain the absence of the trapezium. Also included in the differential would be an osteolytic lesion, but unlikely a result of the straight edge on the first metacarpal base.

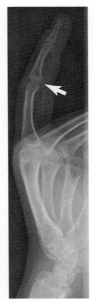

Figure 10-89. ■ Lateral view of a fracture at the volar base of the middle phalanx. Requires 'Zoom' function to see adequately.

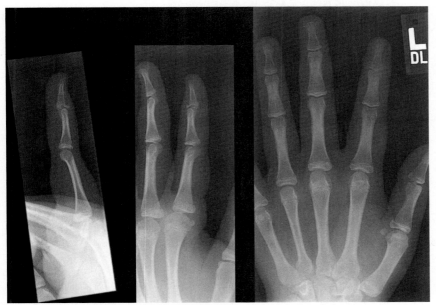

Figure 10-90. ■ Three views: P/A, lateral and oblique. 'Mallet' Fracture, intraarticular, at the base of the index finger DIP.

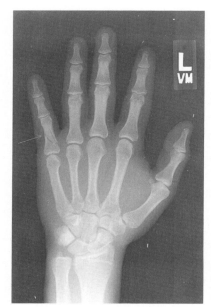

Figure 10-91. ■ P/A view of a fracture of the proximal fifth phalanx.

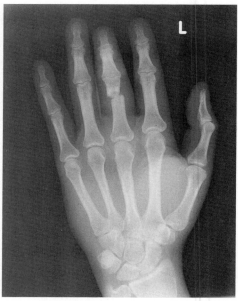

Figure 10-92. ■ P/A view of a fracture of the proximal phalanx of the middle (third or long) finger.

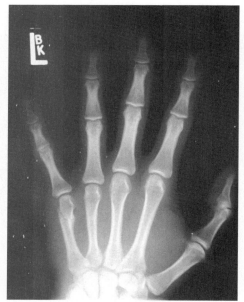

Figure 10-93. ■ P/A view demonstrating a comminuted fracture of the first phalanx on the fifth/small finger.

metacarpals over time, and ultimately, dislocation of multiple joints of the wrist, metacarpals, and digits.

Figures 10-94 to 10-98 depict damage caused by rheumatoid arthritis.

Osteoarthritis is a disease of the larger joints: hips, knees, shoulders, and spine with one exception, the distal phalangeal and proximal interphalangeal joints (PIPs) of the hands. These bumps, known as Heberden's nodes and/or Bouchard's nodes, respectively, develop as calcific spurs as the disease progresses (Figure 10-99).

Bone Density and Dimension

Normal. The individual joints must be carefully evaluated for changes in density that may indicate an occult fracture. Each view must be evaluated and compared with the other PIPs, IPs, and distal interphalangeal joints (DIPs).

Abnormal. Fractures and fracture dislocations, particularly those dislocations and fractures that self-reduce, require carefully studied analysis (Figures 10-100 to 10-109).

Cartilage

Normal. Joint spaces are well maintained.

Abnormal

Soft Tissue

Abnormal. The soft tissue around the metacarpals and phalanges should be equal and demonstrate no evidence of swelling compared with the others on the hand (Figures 10-110 to 10-114).

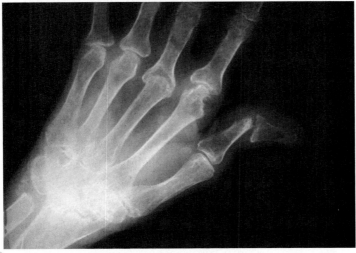

Figure 10-94. ■ P/A view of severe collapse of the wrist and destruction of the MP joints and the IP joint of the thumb in a patient with rheumatoid arthritis.

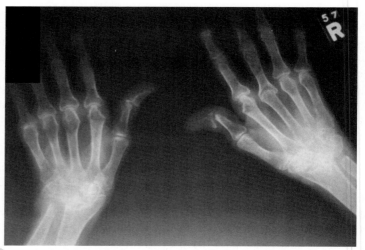

Figure 10-95. ■ Bilateral P/A views of hands with rheumatoid arthritis.

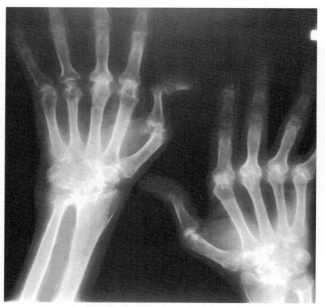

Figure 10-96. ■ Bilateral P/A views of hands with rheumatoid arthritis.

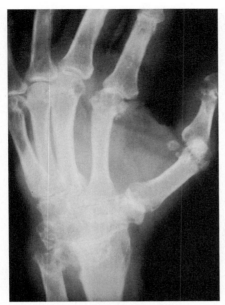

Figure 10-97. ■ Oblique view of subluxation of MP joint of the thumb, erosion and collapse of the carpals and MP joints from rheumatoid arthritis.

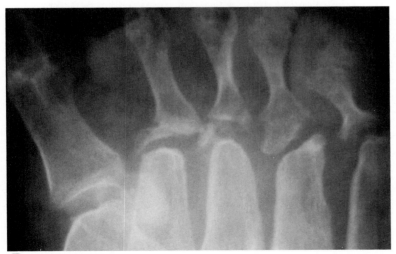

Figure 10-98. ■ P/A view of destruction of the joints in rheumatoid arthritis.

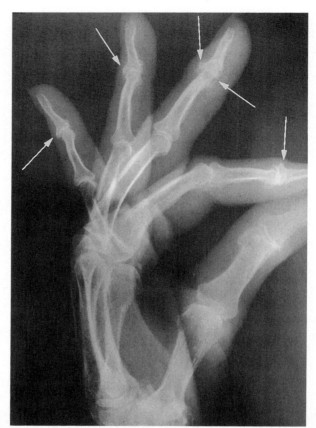

Figure 10-99. ■ Heberden's notes at the base of the distal phalanges dorsally. Indicative of osteoarthritis. *(From Noble J:* Textbook of primary care medicine, *ed 3, St. Louis, Mosby, 2001.)*

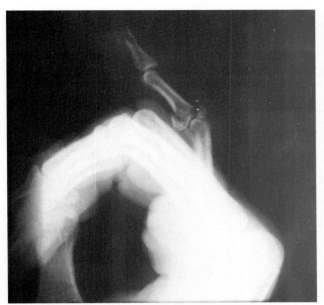

Figure 10-100. ■ Magnified view of fracture of the distal phalanx and intraarticular fracture of the DIP joint in a 28-year-old female softball player who was struck on the end of her small finger by a batted ball.

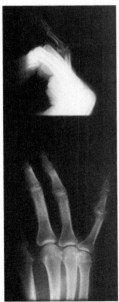

Figure 10-101. ■ Two views of the finger seen in Figure 10-100 isolating views of the two fractures.

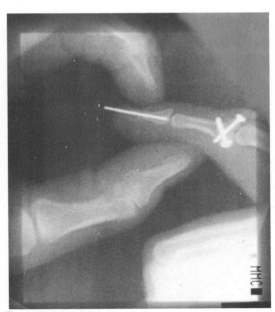

Figure 10-102. ■ Fluoroscopic view of operative pinning of distal fracture and screws to reduce the intraarticular DIP fracture. In young patients, the distal fingers may be crushed or struck directly along the long axis of the bone(s).

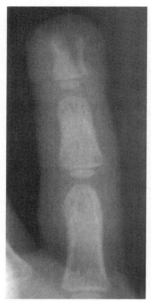

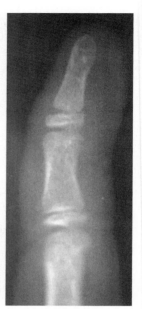

Figure 10-103. ■ Salter-Harris fracture of the distal phalanx and a crush injury.

Figure 10-104. ■ A 15-year-old male athlete with a Salter-Harris Type I injury to the distal phalanx in football.

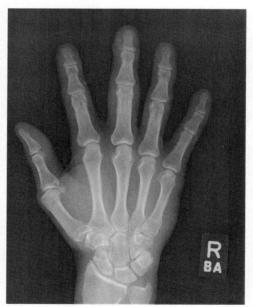

Figure 10-105. ■ P/A view demonstrating a fracture of the long finger/third digit distal phalanx. Note the soft tissue damage at this location.

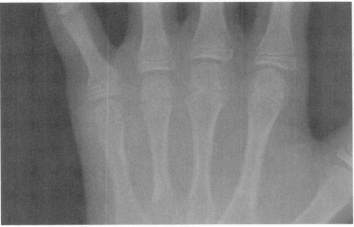

Figure 10-106. ■ P/A view of a Salter-Harris II fracture at the base of the proximal phalanx of the fifth/small finger in a 13-year-old male athlete.

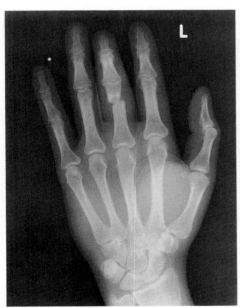

Figure 10-107. ■ P/A view of a fracture of the shaft of the proximal phalanx on the middle/third/long finger.

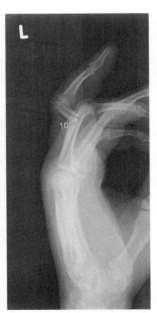

Figure 10-108. ■ Lateral view of a transverse fracture of the proximal phalanx of the third/middle/long finger. Anglulation of the fracture is dorsally to 100 degrees.

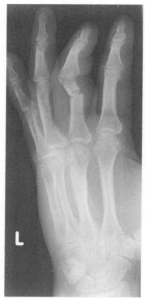

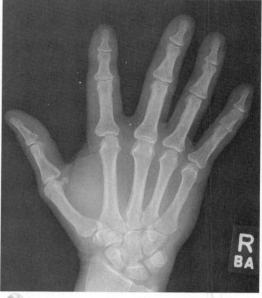

Figure 10-109. ■ Oblique view of a transverse fracture of the proximal phalanx of the third/long/ middle finger.

Figure 10-110. ■ P/A view of right hand.

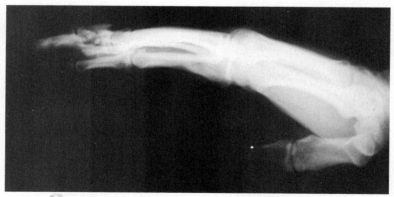

Figure 10-111. ■ Lateral view of man vs. table saw.

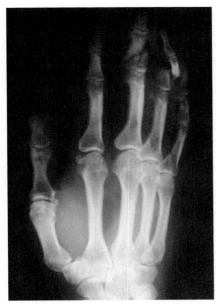

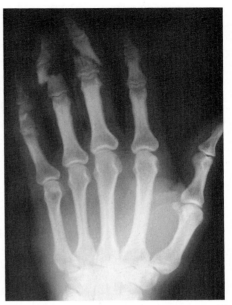

Figure 10-112. ■ Oblique view of man vs. table saw.

Figure 10-113. ■ P/A view of man vs. table saw.

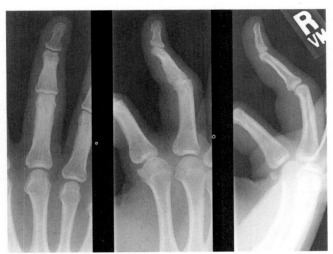

Figure 10-114. ■ Three views of a 'Boutonnière Deformity'. This represents a soft tissue lesion that occurs when the extensor hood mechanism ruptures and subluxes volarly resulting in inability to extend the joint and hyperextension of the distal DIP joint.

Thumb AP and Lateral

Alignment

Normal. The thumb is similar to the other digits, but lacks the middle phalanx. It is the most radial of the fingers and articulates with the trapezium carpal. The thumb is the most mobile of the fingers and can assume the position of opposition to the other metacarpals and digits.

Bone Density and Dimension

Abnormal (Figures 10-115 and 10-116)

Cartilage

Normal. Joint spaces are well maintained.

Abnormal. The absence of joint space between the base of the thumb and the trapezium bone or increased density, or whitening, of the "bone-on-bone" surfaces are abnormal signs. In rheumatoid arthritis, there is a generalized destruction of the connective tissue and cartilage and demineralization of the bones resulting in unstable joints, joint subluxations and/or dislocations, and erosion of the bones around the joints. In the hand and wrist, it tends to be a disease of the carpals, metacarpals, and PIPs (see Figure 10-96).[10]

Soft Tissue

Normal. No evidence of soft tissue swelling or trauma is visible.

Abnormal. The thumb is sensitive to subluxations at all joints, particularly the metacarpophalangeal joint. The ligament damaged most often is the medial (ulnar) side of the metacarpophalangeal joint as a result of tearing of the collateral ligament or avulsion on the insertion of this ligament and is commonly referred to as the "game keeper's thumb." This is verified by a clinical examination that demonstrates inordinate opening at the medial (ulnar) joint when compared with the noninvolved side and on stress views. A "miniarthrogram" (injection of dye) may be used to confirm suspected intraarticular imposition of the torn ligament or avulsed fragment into the joint, which would preclude normal healing (Figure 10-116).

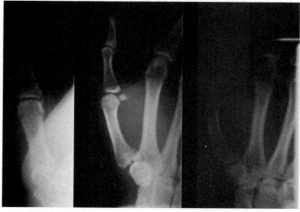

Figure 10-115. ■ A Bennett's fracture is a fracture at the base of the thumb, and the pull of the abductor pollicis longus tendon will displace the portion of the fracture that it is attached to proximally.

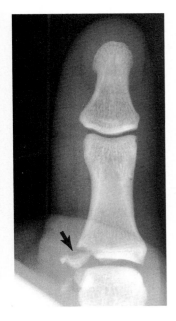

Figure 10-116. ■ Gamekeeper's thumb that reflects a damaged ulnar collateral ligament at the first metacarpophalangeal joint. In an acute injury, as occurs in skiing and falling with the thumb against the ski pole, an avulsion fracture occurs at the base of the first metacarpal. *(From Adam A:* Grainger & Allison's Diagnostic Radiology, *ed 5, Churchill Livingstone, 2008.)*

CASE STUDIES

CASE STUDY A

A/P, Lateral, and oblique views of the wrist on the same set

There are plain films and a contrast film with the same three views shown. A patient fell onto her right arm and hand. Please identify the age within 20 years, and any fractures(s) you identify with and any accompanying angulations. Figure 10-117 and 10-118.

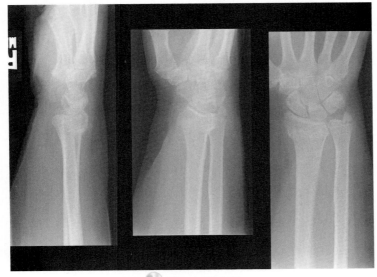

Figure 10-117

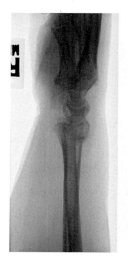
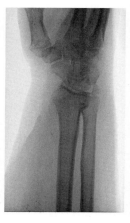
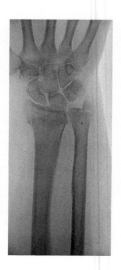

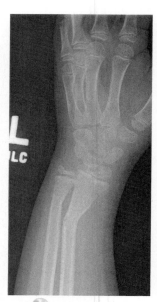

🔘 **Figure 10-118**

CASE STUDY B

A/P, Lateral and Oblique Views of the Wrist

Patient fell onto wrist. Please estimate within 10 years of the age of the patient and any fracture(s) identified by location, angulation, etc. Figures 10-119, 10-120 and 10-121.

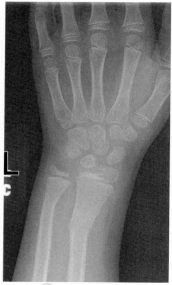

🔘 **Figure 10-119**

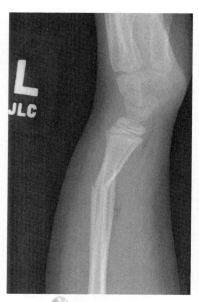

🔘 **Figure 10-120**

🔘 **Figure 10-121**

CASE STUDY C

A 4-year-old male fell onto his right elbow. Two views, AP and lateral and con-trasting views of the left (uninvolved) elbow. Figures 10-122, 10-123, 10-124 and 10-125.

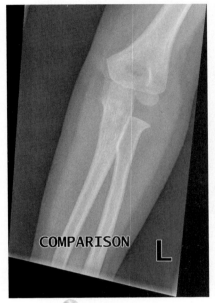

Figure 10-122

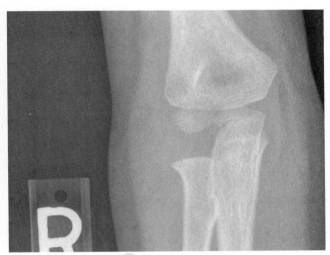

Figure 10-123

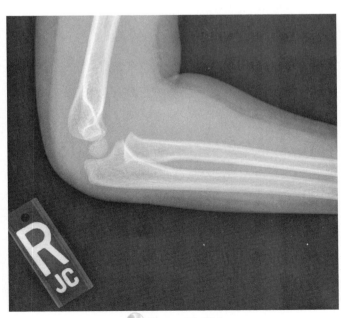

Figure 10-124

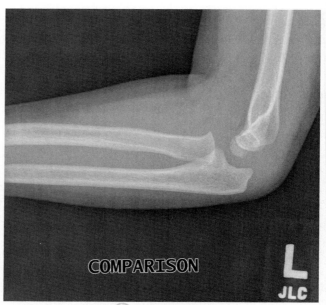

Figure 10-125

REFERENCES

1. Rockwood CA Jr, Green DP, Bucholz RW, *Fractures in adults*, ed 3, New York, 1996, Lippincott Co.
2. Resnick D, Niwayama G, *Diagnosis of bone and joint disorders*, ed 2, 1988, Philadelphia, London, W/B Saunders.
3. Resnick D, Niwayama G, *Diagnosis of bone and joint disorders*, ed 2, 1988, Philadelphia, London, W/B Saunders.
4. Resnick D, Niwayama G, *Diagnosis of bone and joint disorders*, ed 2, 1988, Philadelphia, London, W/B Saunders.
5. Greenspan A, *Orthopedic radiology*, ed 2, 1992, New York, Raven Press.
6. Swain J, *Personal communication from patient in clinic*, Nampa, Idaho 2006.
7. Mason ML, Some Observations on Fractures of the Head of the Radius With a Review of One Hundred Cases. *British Journal of Surgery* 1954 Sept; 47(172): 123 – 132
8. Greenspan A, Orthopedic Radiology, Second Edition, 1992, Raven Press, New York, Pg 5.36
9. Greenspan A, Orthopedic Radiology, Second Edition, 1992, Raven Press, New York, Pg 5.27
10. Greenspan A, Orthopedic Radiology, Second Edition, 1992, Raven Press, New York, Pg 4.14
11. Footnote: Rockwood CA Jr, Green DP, Bucholz RW, Fractures in Adults, Third Edition, Lippincott Co, New York, Chapter 8, Pg 568.
12. Footnote: Netter FH, The Ciba Collection of Medical Illustrations, Volume 8, Musculoskeletal System, Ciba-Geigy Corp, Summit, New Jersey, Pg 66.
13. Rockwood CA Jr, Green DP, Bucholz RW, Fractures in Adults, ed 3, Lippincott Co, New York, Chapter 8, Pg 581.
14. Rockwood CA Jr, Green DP, Bucholz RW, Fractures in Adults, ed 3, Lippincott Co, New York, Chapter 8, Pg 581.
15. Rockwood CA Jr, Green DP, Bucholz RW, Fractures in Adults, ed 3, Lippincott Co, New York, Chapter 8, Pg 580.
16. Rockwood CA Jr, Green DP, Bucholz RW, Fractures in Adults, ed 3, Lippincott Co, New York, Chapter 8, Pg 580.
17. Trumble T: *Avascular Necrosis of the Lunate*: http://www.orthop.washington.edu/uw/kienbocksdisease/tabID__3349/ItemID__275/PageID__1/Articles/Default.aspx Accessed June 18, 2008.
18. Light TR, Ogden DA. The Anatomy of metaphyseal Torus fractures. Clinical Orhopedics 1984: 188: 103 – 111.
19. Resnick D, Niwayama G, *Diagnosis of bone and joint disorders*, Second Edition 1988, W/B Saunders Co, Philadelphia, London, etc, Pg 6.
20. Greenspan A, Orthopedic Radiology, Second Edition, 1992, Raven Press, New York, Pg 6.1.
21. Rockwood CA Jr, Green DP, Bucholz RW, *Fractures in Adults*, ed 3, New York, 1996, Lippincott Co.

11 Magnetic Resonance Imaging

INTRODUCTION

Remarks

Plain film radiographs are able to produce an image of bone by blocking x-rays as they travel through the body. X-ray films therefore are best at visualizing bone. In contrast, magnetic resonance imaging (MRI) is able to depict soft tissues with great accuracy and allows us to "see" soft tissues and bone within the body. Please refer to Chapter 3 for an explanation of how MRI works.

The purpose of this chapter is to demonstrate how we can use MRI in rehabilitation practice to better understand the patient's present condition and his or her prognosis. This chapter demonstrates the use of MRI in the knee. With a thorough knowledge of the anatomy of the human body, the principles demonstrated in this chapter can be used for evaluating MRI images of other body regions.

There is a wealth of information about a patient's condition that can be found in an MRI.

MRIs of the knee will be used to demonstrate the usefulness of MRI in clinical practice.

MRI can add a tremendous amount to our understanding of pathologic conditions. This form of nonionizing imaging can produce high quality images of bone and soft tissue. It is the imaging of choice for soft tissue and the combination of T1 studies, emphasizing anatomy, and T2, emphasizing contrast between tissues, such as a signal contrast as the result of swelling around damaged tissues provides additional information to the clinician. Bone marrow edema (BME) visible as a change in signal intensity within the bone after recent trauma is a

OBJECTIVES

1. Demonstrate the ability to orient to the anatomic location of the MRI images.
2. Identify common anatomic structures on an MRI image.
3. Demonstrate the ability to differentiate between normal and pathologic anatomic images and/or findings.

dramatic example of the power of this modality. MRI studies of the knee are an augmentation to the plain films. The strengths and advantages of employing a technique that is nonionizing and is suited for demonstrating pathologic changes in connective tissue, such as ligaments, tendons, and cartilage, make MRI imaging the most frequently ordered imaging modality for the knee after a regular x-ray series.[1-3] MRI images add much to our understanding of disease processes of the knee, including arthritides, infections, neoplasms, drug effects, and surgical interventions. Trauma to the ligamentous and cartilaginous tissue that stabilize the knee joint is best visualized by this modality. However, it is worth repeating that the preponderance of ligamentous and cartilaginous damage to the knee can be diagnosed by taking a careful history and performing a focused, organized physical examination.[1] Imaging, when used correctly, confirms the diagnosis and defines the extent of the damage to the articular and/or ligamentous structures. The cost of this modality is significantly greater than conventional x-ray films.

VIEWS

Inherent to all understanding of imaging is the thorough knowledge of the anatomy of the structure being imaged. In standard x-ray films, the bony anatomy is the focus; however, MRI studies cut through the soft tissue in 3-mm slices in several planes, including sagittal, tangential, coronal, and axial, providing exquisite detail of the nonbony structures. A progressive appreciation of what is normal contrast between various tissue densities during multiple slices and the consequences to the images during the manipulation of the variables (time to echo, time to repetition, fat suppression, etc.) is the basis of accurate interpretation of this modality. Suspected pathologic conditions will have been identified by the examining or referring practitioner. The focus is on the soft tissues, including ligaments, menisci, hyaline cartilage and subchondral bone, bursae, and any pathologic soft tissue (hematoma, tumors, etc.). The MRI image, as in plain films, may occasionally be diagnostic by what is *not* visualized, as in an absent anterior cruciate ligament (ACL) when the appropriate "cut" is examined. It is beyond the scope of our introductory effort here to provide more than general information concerning the normal cuts and scope of pathologic findings, but an introduction to some of the more common pathologic conditions will be demonstrated and the techniques used to achieve them identified.

Sagittal Orientation

The sagittal view will demonstrate planes that move from side to side throughout the knee.

Coronal Orientation

The coronal view will demonstrate planes that move from front to back throughout the structure.

Axial Orientation

The axial view will demonstrate planes that move through the knee from proximal to distal.

EVALUATION OF THE KNEE

Menisci

It is accepted that MRI is 90% to 95% accurate in the diagnosis of torn menisci in the hands of an expert interpreter, but much lower in less experienced radiologists.[4] The T1 sequence using sagittal and coronal slices is the sequence of choice for evaluating menisci (Figures 11-1 and 11-2).[3]

Moving from the more superficial toward the intercondylar notch, the menisci appear first as a dark (fibrocartilage) anterior-posterior band in the joint, slightly thicker in the anterior and posterior ends than in the middle, a "bow tie" sign.[5] The first two visible cuts of the meniscus should share this appearance. The absence of the bow tie sign was 88% accurate for a tear in one study.[5] As the slices move more medially, toward the notch, the menisci appear only in the anterior and posterior portions of the joint and are shaped like "wedges" or "doorstops" with the anterior horn of the medial meniscus approximately one half of the size of the posterior horn and the lateral horns approximately equal in size.[6] Identification of a tear in the meniscus depends upon the particular slice being evaluated and understanding what is normal for that slice depth (Figures 11-3 to 11-5). For example, the more superficial view of the meniscus may demonstrate the absence of the midsubstance of the band, indicating that the meniscus has a tear that has been displaced medially toward or into the intercondylar notch where it will appear where there should be no meniscal substance. The dark appearance of the meniscal fragment (it is fibrocartilage) may give the appearance of a "double posterior cruciate ligament (PCL)" in the notch (the PCL is a dense ligament and also dark).[3] The bow tie sign should appear on two sequential slices,[7] and the

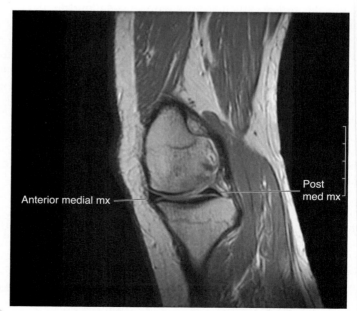

Figure 11-1. ■ A sagittal cut lateral to medial, lateral to the notch.

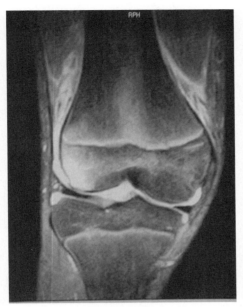

Figure 11-2. ■ A coronal cut of an MRI demonstrating an ACL tear. *(Courtesy of © Kevin Shea, MD, Boise, Idaho.)*

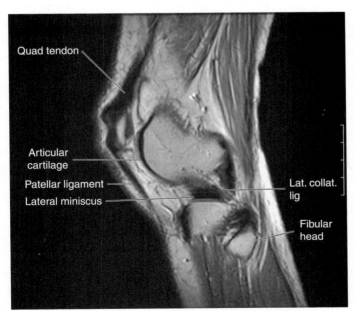

Figure 11-3. ■ This sagittal cut of an MRI lateral to medial demonstrates visible structures as labeled.

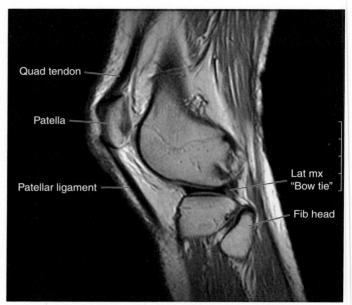

Figure 11-4. ■ This MRI sagittal cut progressing deeper into the knee shows a "bow tie" shape of the lateral meniscus at this depth.

third slice should be wedge shaped. Three sequential bow ties indicate a discoid meniscus or a displaced fragment. Absence of the anterior and posterior wedges on the most medial slice may indicate a discoid meniscus. Tears of the anterior or posterior horns may show as "notches" in the substance of the wedge, an abnormally small wedge, or a blunted wedge as a result of a truncated narrow portion of the wedge where a tear has occurred and been displaced or folded.[3] When the anterior horn of the lateral meniscus (anterior and posterior should be approximately equal in size) is significantly larger than the posterior horn or wedge, it may indicate that a portion of the meniscus has been folded or displaced anteriorly. The tear may appear as a split in the substance of the meniscus (Figure 11-6), a "truncated" wedge as compared with the anterior or posterior section (Figure 11-7), or it may appear as a difference in the density of the substance of the meniscus (Figures 11-8 to 11-10).

Anterior Cruciate Ligament

Normal

The ACL is a wide band of ligamentous tissue about 4 mm thick anterior to posterior. It is less than half the strength of the PCL and appears as a relatively broad band made up of two distinct bundles: the anterior and posterior bundles. The signal of the PCL is darker (more dense) relative to the ACL. The

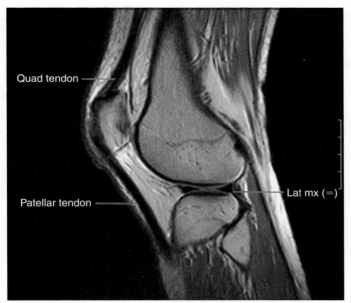

Figure 11-5. ■ Sagittal cut MRI of a bucket handle tear appearing as a split in the meniscus.

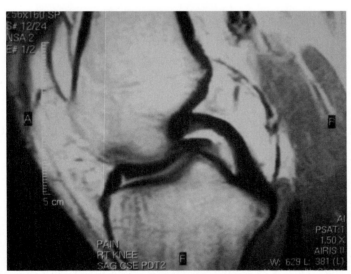

Figure 11-6. ■ Sagittal cut MRI of the knee, lateral compartment just lateral to the notch. Note the wedge appearance of the lateral meniscus. At the depth of this slice the meniscus appears as two separate wedge shaped structures and are referred to as the anterior horn and posterior horn. (*Courtesy of Andrew Curran, MD, Nampa, Idaho*).

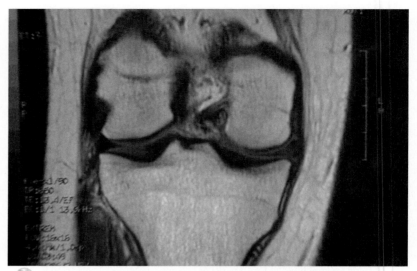

Figure 11-7. ■ A coronal cut MRI of a torn meniscus. *(Courtesy of Andrew Curran, MD, Nampa, Idaho.)*

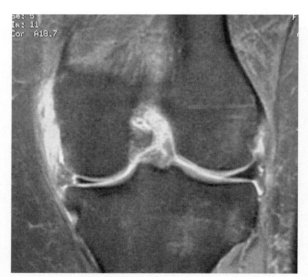

Figure 11-8. ■ A sagittal cut MRI of the posterior horn of a torn meniscus. *(Courtesy of Andrew Curran, MD, Nampa, Idaho.)*

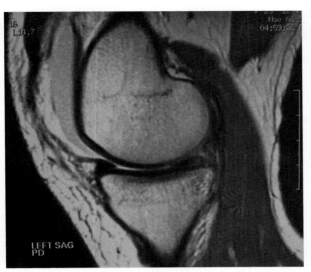

Figure 11-9. ■ **A sagittal cut MRI of a torn posterior horn of the medial meniscus.** Note the tear communicates with the edge of the meniscus. *(Courtesy of Andrew Curran, MD, Nampa, Idaho.)*

ACL connects the posterior lateral corner of the medial femoral condyle in the intercondylar notch with the superior surface of the tibia at the anterior tibial eminence or spine running slightly medially from its proximal attachment to its distal attachment. The cruciates are best evaluated with sagittal, coronal, and axial slices in both the T1 and T2 techniques, but the T2 images are considered more sensitive.[3] The interrater accuracy of MRI evaluation for a torn ACL has been shown to vary significantly between radiologists involved in the same study, from 50% to 82% accuracy.[8] However, other studies have claimed accuracy levels of 90% to 95% in acute, full-thickness tears.[3] The clinical standard is the Lachman's test, and the gold standard for diagnostic accuracy is direct visualization via arthroscopy.

The ACL is easily distinguished from the PCL, which is more dense (darker) on the T1 study. When viewing the specific cut that demonstrates the ACL, the proximal/femoral attachment of the PCL is obscured. The ACL parallels the roof of the intercondylar notch (Blumensaat's line), but does not touch this line (Figures 11-11 to 11-15).[9] If a reconstructed ACL graft is in contact with Blumensaat's line and/or is deflected by the condyle, it is diagnostic of impingement of the graft from inaccurate placement of the graft attachment tunnel(s) (Figure 11-15).[9] If the entire PCL, including the proximal portion, is visible in the cut that normally would demonstrate the ACL, or the proximal portion of the PCL is deflected ("wavy" PCL), the ACL is deficient or torn, as shown in Figure 11-18.

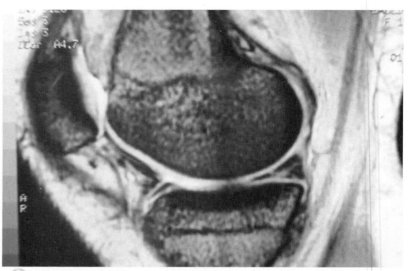

Figure 11-10. ■ Sagittal cut MRI of the knee demonstrating the tear of the posterior horn of the meniscus. Note that the changes in signal—light area—communicates with the inferior periphery of the meniscus indicating a tear. *(Courtesy of Andrew Curran, MD, Nampa, Idaho.)*

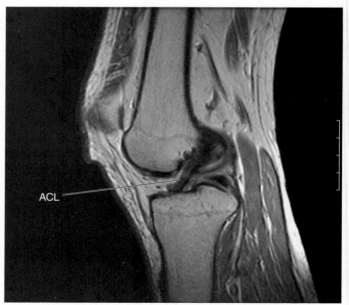

Figure 11-11. ■ **This image continues deeper into the knee with the ACL appearing more as a broad band.** Note that the ACL does not appear as dark (dense) as the PCL.

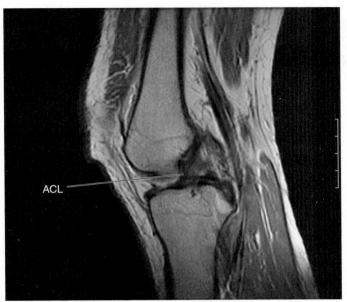

Figure 11-12. ■ Sagittal cut MRI in the notch of the knee demonstrating a lack of ACL, which should be clearly visible as a broad, thin band of tissue running diagonally in the notch.

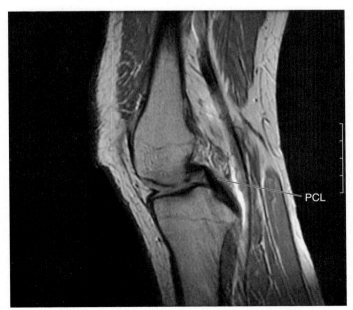

Figure 11-13. ■ The more medial PCL appears as a dark dense band running inferiorly from the medial wall of the notch to the posterior proximal mid tibia. It should appear medially from the ACL.

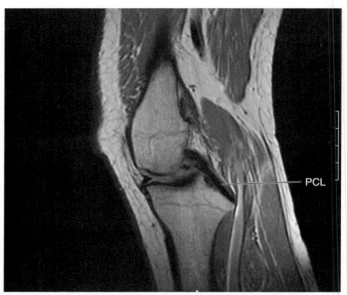

Figure 11-14. ■ **T1 sagittal view of a normal knee.** Note the straight dark structure of the posterior cruciate ligament and the obvious femoral and posterior tibial attachments. *(From Recht MP, Kramer J: MR imaging of the postoperative knee: a pictorial essay,* Radiographics 22:765-774, 2002.)

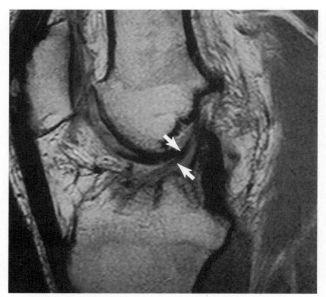

Figure 11-15. ■ **ACL graft impingement in a 36 year old woman.** This cut should show the broad ACL, but instead the PCL is visible through remnants of the ACL. *(From Recht MP, Kramer J: Magnetic Resonance Imaging of the postoperative knee: a pictorial essay,* Radiographics, 22:765-774, 2002.)

Abnormal

The signs of a torn ACL are:

1. Direct visualization of the ACL discontinuity in the sagittal and axial planes was the most sensitive at 95%. Specificity was 85%.[10]
2. Complete nonvisualization in any imaging plane was a specific sign for a complete ACL tear, but was less sensitive and less accurate.
3. The failure of the fascicles of the ACL to parallel the Blumensaat's line was sensitive at 74% to 84% for injury to the ACL.[9]
4. A buckled PCL with the concavity posteriorly on the sagittal MRI images.[3]
5. Weighted sequences were associated with greater sensitivity, specificity, and accuracy than were T1 sequences with false negatives at 0%.
6. An irregular or wavy contour of the anterior margin of the ligament, high signal intensity (brightness) within the ligament on T2, and discontinuity of the substance of the ACL.[10]

Additional signs of the compromise of the ACL are an avulsion of the anterior tibial spine and osseous contusions (as evidenced by an increased (bright) signal relative to the rest of the surrounding bone, (BME) on the T2 images (1) in the posterior lateral femoral condyle or (2) an increased signal in the anterior femoral condyle and anterior proximal tibial spine from hyperextension, as seen in Figure 11-16.[3]

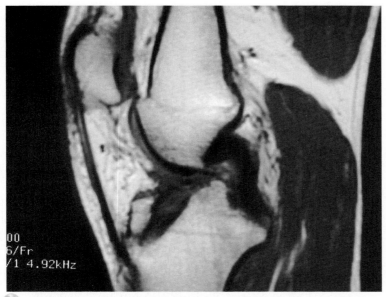

Figure 11-16. ▪ **Sagittal view of the knee fails to show an intact ACL ligament.** Sagittal cut demonstrating a PCL and darkened region/ signal on the femoral condyle that may be bone marrow edema (BME) from a recent trauma. Note "Wavy PCL in this slice. The absence of the ACL and the deflection seen on the PCL indicate a torn ACL. *(From Adam A: Grainger & Allison's* Diagnostic Radiology, *5e, Churchill Livingstone, 2008.)*

Posterior Cruciate Ligament

Normal

The PCL is a dark, dense ligament best identified on MRI in the sagittal cut. It is partially visible with the ACL as a dark, dense structure connecting the posterior tibial eminence to the medial wall of the medial condyle within the femoral notch. It is first encountered as you move lateral to medial through the knee in the sagittal slices through the notch and is partially visible with the ACL. The rest of the PCL should be visible as you move to the next one or two slices laterally.

Abnormal

Refer to Figure 11-6. This view shows a bucket handle tear of the medial meniscus and demonstrates a normal PCL. Contrast the normal PCL in Figure 11-13 with the wavy PCL avulsion shown in Figure 11-18. The PCL is best viewed in a T2 sagittal study. It initially appears with the ACL, with which it partially overlaps, and in the next more medial image as a separate ligament.

The PCL is most frequently injured during direct trauma to the anterior tibia forcing it in a posterior direction relative to the femur and placing direct stress on the PCL fibers. Examples are: skiing into a stump, striking the dashboard with a flexed knee in a motor vehicle accident, or a hyperextension injury in sports, such as being tackled straight on into the tibia while the foot is weight

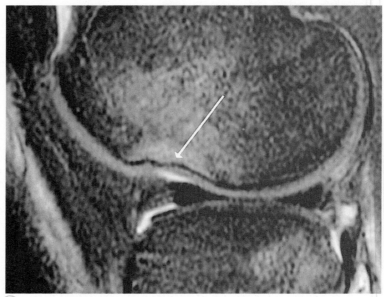

Figure 11-17. ■ Sagittal cut, MRI, demonstrating an osteochondral defect in the lateral condyle. Arrow points to the defect and the surrounding BME indicating that this is a recent injury. *(From DeLee JC, Drez D:* DeLee and Drez's Orthopaedic Sports Medicine, *2nd ed, Saunders, Philadelphia, 2003.)*

bearing and fixed. The PCL is denser and twice as strong as the ACL and appears dark or black on the T1 sagittal cuts when compared with the broader, less dense ACL.[3] Tears of the PCL are seen as a discontinuity of the entire substance of the fibers in a complete tear, as an avulsion of the tibial or femoral attachment of the PCL with increased signal in the specific bony attachment demonstrating bone marrow edema (BME) as in Figure 11-17, or in a partial tear as an increased signal within the fibers. In a complete tear, the PCL should show a gap between the more dense proximal and distal remnants and/or a retraction of the ligament from the opposite remnant. In a recent, direct trauma injury, confirmation should be found on a T2 sagittal slice demonstrating BME in the anterior proximal tibia.[3]

Collateral Ligaments

Abnormal

MRI best demonstrates a medial collateral ligament (MCL) and/or a lateral collateral ligament (LCL) tear in a coronal series (Figure 11-19). The MCL is a large, thick, extracapsular ligament that spans the entire medial joint and appears dark on a T_2 coronal slice. The slice that demonstrates the LCL runs from the lateral femoral condyle to the fibular head where it inserts with the tendon of the biceps femoris (Figure 11-19 and 11-22). It resists varus stress to the lateral complex on the knee and receives support in varying degrees from the iliotibial band.

Cysts in the joint are fluid-filled sacs that produce a bright signal on the T2-weighted sequences. They can be from meniscal tears, cruciate tears, muscle

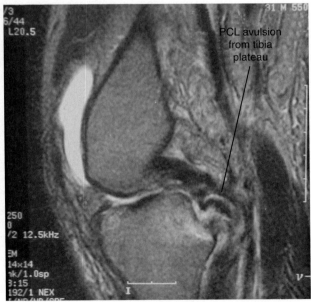

Figure 11-18. ■ Sagittal cut demonstrating a PCL that is avulsed from the tibial insertion. Note the BME indicating that this is a recent injury. *(Courtesy of © Kevin Shae, MD, Boise, Idaho.)*

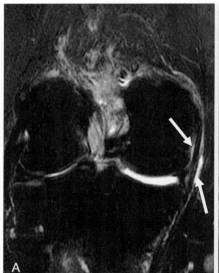

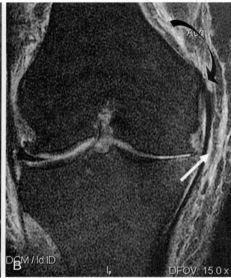

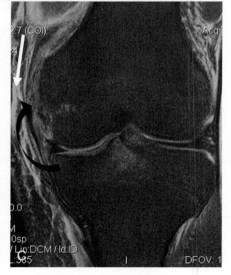

Figure 11-19. ■ **(A)** Coronal T2-weighted MR image with fat saturation shows fluid surrounding the medial collateral ligament (MCL) *(white arrows)* but no evidence of ligament fiber disruption. This appearance is consistent with a first-degree MCL injury in this patient who sustained a sharp blow to the lateral portion of the knee. **(B)** Coronal T2-weighted MR image with fat saturation demonstrates a second-degree MCL injury with fluid surrounding the MCL *(white arrow)* and partial disruption of the fibers of the superior portion of the MCL *(black curved arrow)*. **(C)** Coronal T2-weighted MR image with fat saturation reveals a third degree MCL injury with complete disruption of the proximal MCL *(black curved arrow)* and fluid surrounding the medial ligamentous structures of the knee *(white arrow)*. *(From Beall DP, et al: Magnetic Resonance Imaging of the Collateral Ligaments and the Anatomic Quadrants of the Knee,* Radiologic Clinics of North America - November 2007 *(Vol. 45, Issue 6, Pages 983-1002)*

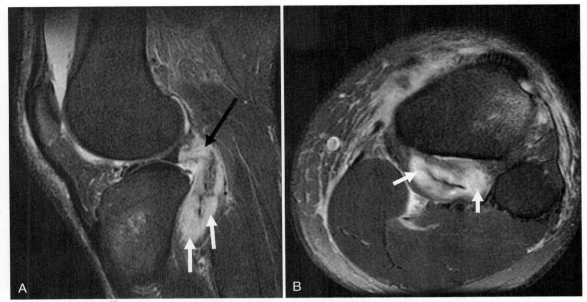

Figure 11-20. ■ **(A)** Sagittal and **(B)** axial T2-weighted MR images with fat saturation show edema *(white arrows in A and B)* surrounding a musculotendinous junction rupture of the popliteus *(black arrow in A)*. *(From Beall DP, et al: Magnetic Resonance Imaging of the Collateral Ligaments and the Anatomic Quadrants of the Knee,* Radiologic Clinics of North America - November 2007 *(Vol. 45, Issue 6, Pages 983-1002)*

tears, or synovial injuries and are visible in slices where they would not normally be found (Figure 11-21).

Osteochondral Defects (OCDs)

Normal

Hyaline cartilage is found in all joints at the bone-to-bone interfaces (Figure 11-21). The hyaline, or articular, cartilage in the knee appears as a dark line contiguous with the distal margins of the femoral condyles, the tibial plateau below the menisci, and the undersurface of the patella. Figure 11-22 is a T2 coronal MRI of a normal knee with labeled structures.

Abnormal

A change in the continuity of this line or a visible defect, a "pothole," seen on the T1- or T2-weighted images indicates an OCD (Figures 11-23 to 11-28). If the change is accompanied by an increased signal in the T2 study in the surrounding bone marrow, BME, the injury is recent in nature. Without the bruising in the adjacent bone marrow, the injury is most likely an older injury. On a T2, fat-saturated image, the hyaline, or articular, cartilage should be black. A break in the continuity of this black line along the bone would indicate an OCD; if the signal is bright where the dark line of hyaline should be continuous, an OCD exists. If it is a recent injury there should be bone marrow edema (BME) visible in the bone surrounding the OCD.

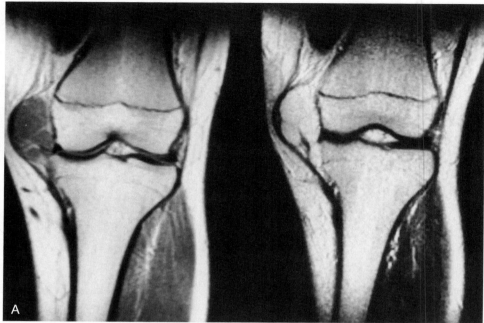

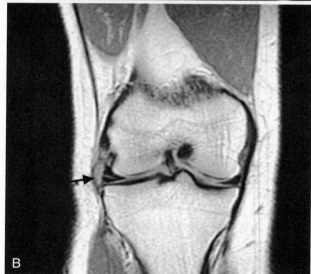

Figure 11-21. ■ Coronal cuts, MRI, demonstrating **A.** Meniscal cyst, dark on one figure and light on other. **B.** Demonstrates horizontal line on the lateral meniscus and a cyst on the lateral aspect of the meniscus. *(A. From Adam A:* Grainger & Allison's Diagnostic Radiology, *5e, Churchill Livingstone, 2008. B. From DeLee JC, Drez D:* DeLee and Drez's Orthopaedic Sports Medicine, *2nd ed, Saunders, Philadelphia, 2003.)*

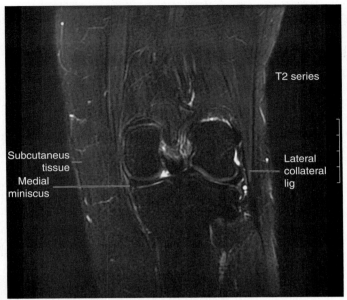

Figure 11-22. ■ Coronal cut, MRI demonstrating the menisci medially and laterally.

Patella

Normal

The patella may be viewed on sagittal, coronal, and axial slices in both the T1- and T2-weighted images. The bone may be evaluated on the T2-weighted images for BME, indicating direct trauma from an impact or fall.

Abnormal

A recent **lateral patellar** dislocation will demonstrate BME, usually on the medial portion of the patella. Trauma to the patella requires a careful review of the articular cartilage on both the underside of the patella with axial and sagittal slices and the area of the **lateral** femoral articular surface impacted by the patella to rule out OCDs.

OCDs may be noted on plain film x-rays on the anteroposterior (AP) and lateral views and MRI on both sagittal and coronal series, as demonstrated in the series of Figures 11-24 to 11-28.

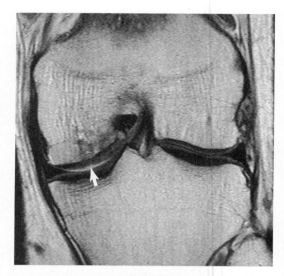

Figure 11-23. ■ **Follow-up evaluation in a 34-year-old woman after osteochondrial autograft transplantation.** Coronal proton density weighted fast spin echo image (3,4000/43 echo train length of 7) demonstrates mild irregularity *(arrowhead)* of the surface of the repair tissue at the transplantation site on the medical femoral condyle. *(From Recht MP, Kramer J:* Magnetic Resonance Imaging of the postoperative knee: a pictorial essay, *Radiographics, 22:765-744, 2002.)*

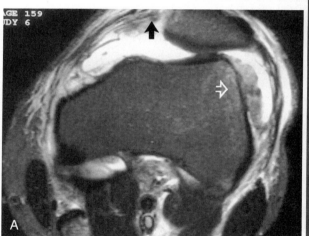

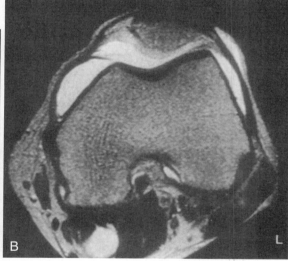

Figure 11-24. ■ **A.** MRI appearance of transient patello-femoral dislocation. Axial STIR image of the knee in a patient who had experienced transient patellar dislocation demonstrates disruption of, and abnormal high signal surrounding the medial patellar retinaculum *(solid arrow).* Oedema in the medial patella and lateral femoral condyle *(open arrow)* represents contusions. There is a moderate joint effusion. The patella remains subluxed. **B.** Contrast Magnetic Resonance Imaging (MRI) Scan of the Knee (axial view) Illustrating a Plica or Medial Shelf. The redundant fold of synovium is seen to the left of the patella as a line of low uptake outlined by contrast within the joint space. (**A.** *From Adam A:* Grainger & Allison's Diagnostic Radiology, *5e, Churchill Livingstone, 2008.* **B.** *From Harris ED, et al:* Kelly's textbook of rheumatology, *7e, Philadelphia, Saunders, 2008.)*

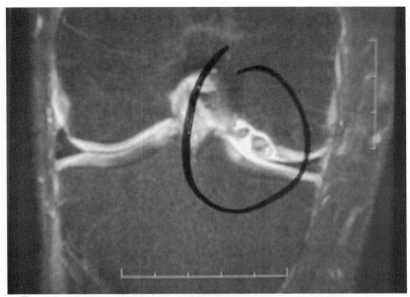

Figure 11-25. ■ This coronal cut MRI demonstrates an OCD and defect in the bone. If there has been a recent injury, the bone around the area will be a different density showing BME. *(Courtesy of Andrew Curran, MD, Nampa, Idaho.)*

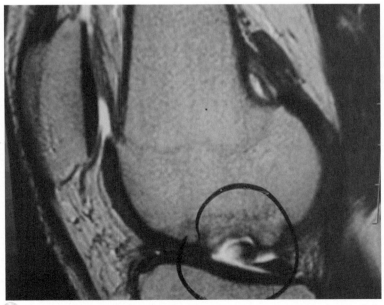

Figure 11-26. ■ This sagittal cut MRI demonstrates an OCD of the medial femoral condyle. *(Courtesy of Andrew Curran, MD, Nampa, Idaho.)*

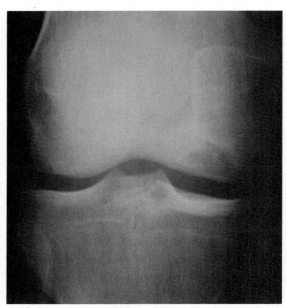

Figure 11-27. ■ **This AP view x-ray film demonstrates an OCD of the medial femoral condyle.** Note the decreased density. *(Courtesy of Andrew Curran, MD, Nampa, Idaho.)*

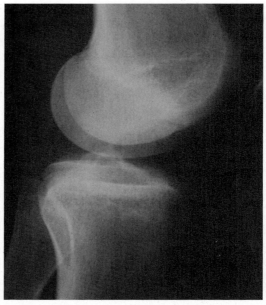

Figure 11-28. ■ **This lateral view x-ray film demonstrates an OCD of the medial femoral condyle.** Note the decreased density.

CASE STUDY A

An adult male arrives in the clinic with a visible lump on the front of his knee anterior and inferior to the patella and inability to fully flex or extend his knee. He describes a vague history with multiple trauma and swelling in the knee. A careful clinical exam reveals a mass on the anterior knee and knee motion limited in the extremes. Motor and sensation are intact and ligaments appear intact. Figures 11-29 to 11-31.

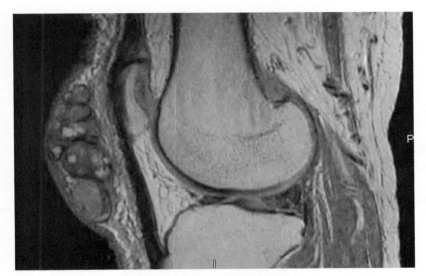

Figure 11-29. ■ MRI studies reveal a lobulated, calcified mass in the prepatellar region on the sagittal T1 and T2 studies and a torn posterior lateral meniscus; note the communication of the tear with the periphery of the meniscus. This is confirmed on the axial cut. The calcified nature of the lobulations confirm that this is not a recent injury.

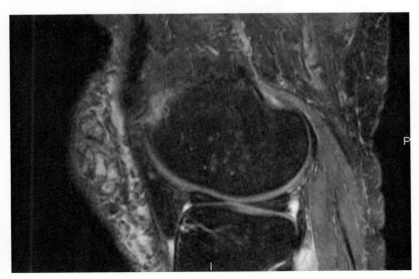

Figure 11-30. ■ MRI studies reveal a lobulated, calcified mass in the prepatellar region on the sagittal T1 and T2 studies and a torn posterior lateral meniscus; note the communication of the tear with the periphery of the meniscus. This is confirmed on the axial cut. The calcified nature of the lobulations confirm that this is not a recent injury.

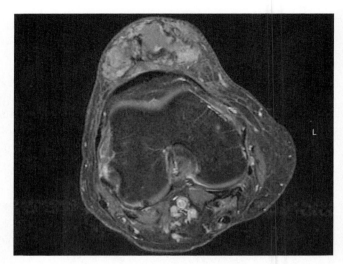

Figure 11-31. ■ MRI studies reveal a lobulated, calcified mass in the prepatellar region on the sagittal T1 and T2 studies and a torn posterior lateral meniscus; note the communication of the tear with the periphery of the meniscus. This is confirmed on the axial cut. The calcified nature of the lobulations confirm that this is not a recent injury.

CASE STUDY B

Athlete with chronic locking, swelling and pain in post medial knee. Figures 11-32 to 11-34. View the following 3 films and determine the patient's problem that causes locking, swelling, and pain.

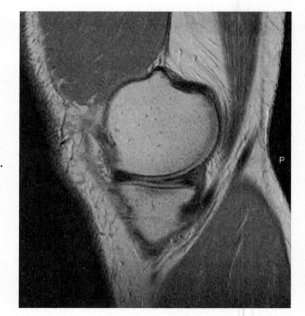

Figure 11-32. ■ T1 sagittal view of the knee.

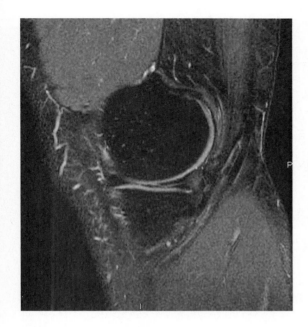

Figure 11-33. ■ **A T2 sagittal view of the knee.**

Our Impressions: The T1 and T2 MRIs reveal a tear in the posterior medial meniscus. The axial view demonstrates a high signal intensity, indicating a cystic formation in the area of the tear.

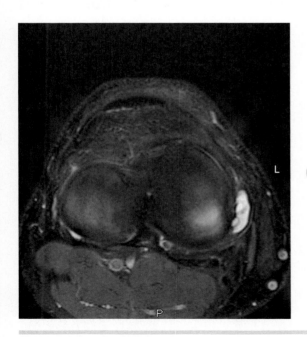

Figure 11-34. ■ **An axial view of the knee.**

CASE STUDY C

A 50-year-old female fell from a hay wagon and sustained injury to knee. Immediate swelling and pain and difficulty bearing weight on knee. Figures 11-35 to 11-37.

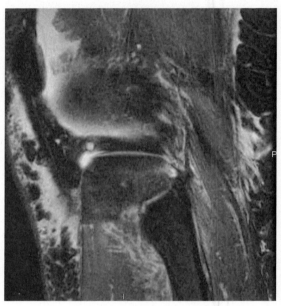

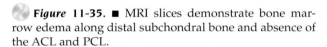 **Figure 11-35.** ■ MRI slices demonstrate bone marrow edema along distal subchondral bone and absence of the ACL and PCL.

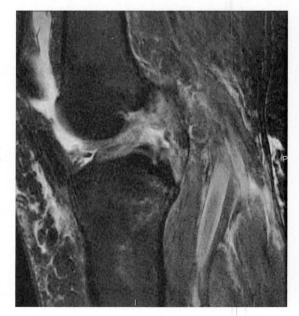

Figure 11-36. ■ MRI slices demonstrate bone marrow edema along distal subchondral bone and absence of the ACL and PCL.

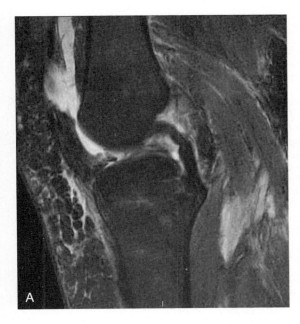

Figure 11-37a. ■ MRI slices demonstrate bone marrow edema along distal subchondral bone and absence of the ACL and PCL.

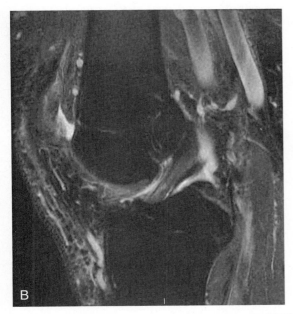

Figure 11-37b. ■ MRI slices demonstrate bone marrow edema along distal subchondral bone and absence of the ACL and PCL. Note the straight ACL on this view of a normal ACL

REFERENCES

1. Tandeter HB, Shvartzman P, Stevens M: Acute knee injuries: use of decision rules for selective radiograph ordering, *Am Fam Phys* 60:4, 1999.
2. Manaster BJ, Ensign MF: Imaging the ligaments of the knee, *Crit Rev Diag Imag* 32:323-366, 1991.
3. Sanders TG, Miller MD: Systematic approach to magnetic resonance imaging interpretation of sports medicine injuries of the knee, *AmJ Sports Med* 33(1):131-148, 2005.
4. Zairul-Nizam AF, Hyzan MY, Gobinder S, et al: The role of preoperative magnetic resonance imaging in internal derangement of the knee, *Med J Malaysia* 55(4):433-438, 2000.
5. Dorsay TA, Helms CA: Bucket-handle meniscal tears of the knee: sensitivity and specificity of MRI signs, *Skel Rad* 32:266-272, 2003.
6. Miller TT, Staron RB, Feldman F, et al: Meniscal position on routine MR imaging of the knee. *Skelet Radiol* 26:424-427, 1997.
7. Chaplin RW, Reeves BE, Pope T: Bucket handle tears of the medial meniscus accompanying a rupture of the ACL, *App Radiol* L34(8):35-37, 2005.
8. Jackson JL, Omalley PG, Koenke K: Evaluation of acute knee pain in primary care, *Ann Intern Med* 139:575-588, 2003.
9. Recht MP, Kramer J: MR imaging of the postoperative knee: a pictorial essay, *Radiographics* 22:765-774, 2002.
10. Lee JK, Yao L, Wirth CR, et al: Anterior cruciate ligament tears: MR imaging compared with arthroscopy and clinical tests, *Radiol* 166:861-864, 1988.

Index